International Perspectives in Critical Care Nursing

Editor

CHRISTI DELEMOS

CRITICAL CARE NURSING CLINICS OF NORTH AMERICA

www.ccnursing.theclinics.com

Consulting Editor
CYNTHIA BAUTISTA

March 2021 • Volume 33 • Number 1

ELSEVIER

1600 John F. Kennedy Boulevard • Suite 1800 • Philadelphia, Pennsylvania, 19103-2899

http://www.theclinics.com

CRITICAL CARE NURSING CLINICS OF NORTH AMERICA Volume 33, Number 1
March 2021 ISSN 0899-5885, ISBN-13: 978-0-323-77634-9

Editor: Kerry Holland
Developmental Editor: Laura Fisher

Critical Care Nursing Clinics of North America (ISSN 0899-5885) is published quarterly by Elsevier Inc., 360 Park Avenue South, New York, NY 10010-1710. Months of issue are March, June, September, and December. Business and Editorial Offices: 1600 John F. Kennedy Blvd., Suite 1800, Philadelphia, PA 19103-2899. Periodicals postage paid at New York, NY and additional mailing offices. Subscription prices are $160.00 per year for US individuals, $576.00 per year for US institutions, $100.00 per year for US students and residents, $206.00 per year for Canadian individuals, $596.00 per year for Canadian institutions, $230.00 per year for international individuals, $596.00 per year for international institutions, $115.00 per year for international students/residents and $100.00 per year for Canadian students/residents. To receive student/resident rate, orders must be accompanied by name of affiliated institution, data of term, and the *signature* of program/residency coordinator on institution letterhead. Orders will be billed at individual rate until proof of status is received. Foreign air speed delivery is included in all *Clinics* subscription prices. All prices are subject to change without notice. **POSTMASTER:** Send address changes to *Critical Care Nursing Clinics of North America*, Elsevier Health Sciences Division, Subscription Customer Service, 3251 Riverport Lane, Maryland Heights, MO 63043. **Customer Service: 1-800-654-2452 (US and Canada); 314-447-8871 (outside US and Canada). Fax: 314-447-8029. E-mail:** JournalsCustomerService-usa@elsevier.com **(for print support) and** JournalsOnlineSupport-usa@elsevier.com **(for online support).**

Reprints. For copies of 100 or more of articles in this publication, please contact the Commercial Reprints Department, Elsevier Inc., 360 Park Avenue South, New York, New York, 10010-1710; Tel.: 212-633-3874, Fax: 212-633-3820, and E-mail: reprints@elsevier.com.

Critical Care Nursing Clinics of North America is covered in *MEDLINE/PubMed (Index Medicus), International Nursing Index, Nursing Citation Index, Cumulative Index to Nursing and Allied Health Literature, and RNdex Top 100.*

Printed in the United States of America.

Contributors

CONSULTING EDITOR

CYNTHIA BAUTISTA, PhD, APRN, FNCS, FCNS
Associate Professor, Egan School of Nursing and Health Studies, Fairfield University, Fairfield, Connecticut, USA

EDITOR

CHRISTI DELEMOS, MS, CNRN, ACNP-BC
President of the World Federation of Neuroscience Nurses, Director of Advanced Practice, UC Davis Health, Sacramento, California, USA

AUTHORS

SHEILA A. ALEXANDER, PhD, RN, FCCM
Associate Professor, Acute and Tertiary Care, School of Nursing, Critical Care Medicine, School of Medicine, University of Pittsburgh, Pittsburgh, Pennsylvania, USA

MARÍA CONSUELO AMAYA-REY, RN, BS, FNP, MSN, PhD
Professor, Nursing Faculty, Universidad Nacional de Colombia, Bogotá, D.C., Colombia

NEAL F. COOK, PhD, MSc, PG Dip Nurse Education, PG Cert, BSc Hons, Dip Aromatherapy, RN, Lecturer/Practice Educator, Specialist Practitioner Adult, PFHEA
Reader, Associate Head of School, School of Nursing, Ulster University, Londonderry, Northern Ireland

TERESA DEFFNER, PhD
Clinical Psychologist, Department of Anesthesiology and Intensive Care Medicine, Jena University Hospital, Jena, Germany

VICKI EVANS, RN
GradDip Neuroscience, GradDip Nursing Management, Vice President, World Federation of Neuroscience Nurses; Clinical Nurse Consultant, Neuroscience, Royal North Shore Hospital, Sydney, Australia

ANGELA GNANADURAI, MSc (N), PhD(N)
Principal, Jubilee Mission College of Nursing, Jubilee Mission Medical College and Research Institute, Thrissur, Kerala, India

KAREN CZARINA S. ILANO, RN, SCRN
Member, Critical Care Nurses Association of the Philippines, Inc., Quezon City, Philippines

VIRGINIA SOTO LESMES, RN, MSN, PhD
Professor, Nursing Faculty, Universidad Nacional de Colombia, Bogotá, D.C., Colombia

RUDOLF CYMORR KIRBY P. MARTINEZ, PhD, MA, RN
Professorial Lecturer, Graduate School of Nursing, Arellano University Juan Sumulong Campus, Assistant Professor, College of Nursing, San Beda University, Manila, Philippines

PETER NYDAHL, RN, MScN, PhD
Nursing Research, Department of Anaesthesiology and Intensive Care Medicine, University Hospital Schleswig-Holstein, Kiel, Germany

STEFANY ORTEGA-PEREZ, RN, MSc, PhD
Assistant Professor, Nursing Department, Universidad del Norte, Barranquilla, Colombia

ANNE PREECE, RN, RM, BSc(Hons)
Clinical Nursing Studies Specialist Practitioner, MSc. Head Injury Clinical Nurse Specialist, Neurosciences, Recent Past President, British Association Neuroscience Nurses, Queen Elizabeth Hospital, Edgbaston, Birmingham, United Kingdom

MARIA ISABELITA C. ROGADO, MA, RN
Professorial Lecturer, Graduate School of Nursing, Arellano University Juan Sumulong Campus, Manila, Philippines; President, Critical Care Nurses Association of the Philippines, Inc., Quezon City, Philippines

DIANA JEAN F. SERONDO, RN, SCRN, NVRN-BC
Secretary, Critical Care Nurses Association of the Philippines, Inc., Quezon City, Philippines

GIL P. SORIANO, MHPEd, RN
Assistant Professor, Graduate School Wesleyan University - Philippines, Cabanatuan City, Nueva Ecija, Philippines; Assistant Professor, College of Nursing, San Beda University, Manila, Philippines

SALLY YOUNG, RN, BSc(Hons)
Nursing, Subarachnoid Clinical Nurse Specialist, Neurosciences, Queen Elizabeth Hospital, Edgbaston, Birmingham, United Kingdom

Contents

> This integrative review presents the most recent and relevant critical care nursing research publications in the United States. A comprehensive search identified publications on the topics of delirium; early mobility; communication; palliative care; tele–intensive care unit; care bundle implementation; and prevention, detection, and early management of infection. The evidence is summarized for each of these topics, as well as other research, with suggestions and guidance for end users.

> Each year, millions of people suffer traumatic brain injury (TBI). It is not inherent to any country or group of people. It occurs as a result of falls, combat situations, sports injury, schoolyard playgrounds, and car accidents. It does not discriminate with age or status. Cost implications for health care settings and individuals are substantial. Management requires prompt neurologic assessment by a highly specialized multidisciplinary team of neuroscience practitioners. It is important to understand normal brain anatomy and physiology to identify what is unusual or abnormal. Keen observational skills and constant questioning aid in early detection of neurologic deterioration.

> Diaries are written for patients in intensive care units by staff and relatives, especially when patients experience a disorder of their consciousness, such as delirium. Diary entries are written in common language, describing the situation of the patient. The diary can be read by the patient and the family and support the coping and understanding of what happened. It can function as a tool for supporting communication about different experiences and views of critical illness.

> The risk of rebleeding is greatest between 2 and 12 hours and is associated with increased risk of mortality and long-term dependent survival. Aneurysms should be secured within 48 hours of diagnosis. However, delays occur because of diagnosis and transfer of patients. Ninety-six hours is the

current time it can take until treatment. The challenges for this service continue to be access to and sharing of diagnostic imaging, repatriation back to district general hospitals to continue treatment (eg, for rehabilitation), access to neurorehabilitation, and access to psychological and neurocognitive support.

Critical care nursing and medicine have evolved significantly over the past few decades. Critical care in India began the major urban hospitals and has not yet become established in rural health care facilities. The formation of Indian critical care nursing and medical societies led to emerging regular conferences, updates, continuing nursing and medical education, workshops, and training programs for the further training of nurses and doctors. Future challenges include development of guidelines and consolidation of research activities on the outcome of patients with critical illness. This article describes the organization and practice of critical care nursing in India.

This article provides a brief background on critical care nursing in the Philippines, its trend on current practice, and its implication and future direction. An overview is given on the milieu and processes inherent in the critical care unit with the intensive care unit setup taken as its exemplar. The roles and responsibilities of critical care nurses within these units and nature of common issues within their practice is explored. The need for training in communication skills, conflict resolution, and palliative care is implied for these nurses to fully fulfill their roles as collaborative clinician and active patient advocate.

Although the Glasgow Coma Scale has made a positive contribution to the care of people with neurologic orders, variance exists in its understanding and application secondary to inconsistency in guidelines, their interpretation, and the educational approach to the use of the tool. This fragmentation has been evidenced to result in variances in practice, some potentially harmful. Also, recent evidence demonstrates human factors, such as distress, have not been addressed within such education and guidelines for use. An opportunity now exists to take a new, unified approach to education and standards for use of the tool, framed within a person-centered context.

Traumatic brain injury and stroke are the leading causes of death and disability in Latin American and Caribbean countries. Specific characteristics, models of health care systems, and risk factors may influence the patient's outcome in this region. Relevant literature suggest that important delay problems exist in seeking care, reaching care, and receiving care in patients with acute neurologic injuries. Minimizing the time lost before care can be provided are vital to reduce the morbidity, long-term disability, and improved survival.

International Perspectives in Critical Care Nursing

CRITICAL CARE NURSING CLINICS OF NORTH AMERICA

SERIES OF RELATED INTEREST

Nursing Clinics of North America
http://www.nursing.theclinics.com

THE CLINICS ARE AVAILABLE ONLINE!
Access your subscription at:
www.theclinics.com

Preface: Global Intensive Care Management Strategies

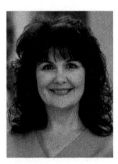

Christi DeLemos, MS, CNRN, ACNP-BC
Editor

Nearly 70 years ago, the concept of critical care units was introduced by Dr William McClenahan to improve the delivery of care for severely ill patients.[1] These changes were fueled by surgical advances that created patients with fast changing needs requiring dedicated staff. Within 5 years, the intensive care unit had been adopted by 90% of large US-based hospitals. Dedicated critical care beds represent 2% to 6% of all hospital beds in developed countries.[2] Nurses working in critical care built on World War II experience and began to develop structure and standards to support critical care nursing.[2] Today, critical care nurses are educated in evidence-based protocolized care that optimizes functional outcome and survival.

Internationally, critical care nursing is an organized field with an established framework that supports specialty education and certification. These standards ensure that nursing care delivered optimizes the chance for recovery. In developed countries with high income, expertise in technology, mechanical ventilation, and titration of vasoactive drips is defining skills. Critical care in low-resource settings calls on the ingenuity and medical experience of nurses rather than the technology we have become so accustomed to. Development of formal triage systems and bedside skill to recognize sudden, serious reversible disease using basic resuscitation techniques is important.[2]

Despite technological advances in imaging and monitoring techniques, neurologic assessment remains the cornerstone of effective detection and treatment of neurologic disease. Accurate neurologic assessment allows medical providers to detect subtle changes over time that may herald increasing injury to the nervous system or signs of recovery. Over the past decade, health care providers have been bombarded with training aimed at managing increasingly complex technology to measure intracranial pressure (ICP), velocity of blood flow in the brain, and brain tissue oxygenation with less time dedicated to sound examination techniques. This technology-focused approach to care was challenged by Chestnut and colleagues,[3] who compared a simple neurologic examination to an intensive ICP monitor-driven approach to care. The

Crit Care Nurs Clin N Am 33 (2021) ix–x
https://doi.org/10.1016/j.cnc.2020.10.008
0899-5885/21/© 2020 Published by Elsevier Inc.

BEST-TRIP study was conducted in intensive care units in Bolivia and Ecuador, where ICP monitoring was not considered a standard of care.[3] Three hundred twenty-four subjects were randomly assigned to one of 2 protocols: ICP goal-directed management to maintain the ICP less than 20 or a treatment protocol based on imaging and clinical examination alone. The primary outcome was survival and functional outcome at 3 and 6 months after injury.

The study found no significant difference in the outcome of those who used expensive monitoring devices and those whose care was directed by imaging and clinical examination alone. Even with access to advanced imaging and monitoring, we must rely on the skill of nurses and other health care providers to recognize the signs of clinical deterioration.

This study underscores the value of developing an educational program aimed at basic bedside skills as a strategy in the global effort to reduce morbidity and mortality associated with traumatic brain injury and neurologic disease.

This issue reviews a range of intensive care management strategies from across the world. When available, monitoring equipment and careful measurement of progress with diagnostics are desirable. But it does not replace the skillful examination of the bedside nurse. The most promising strategy for effective treatment of neurologic disorders in patients across the world is early recognition and appropriate medical care.[4]

Christi DeLemos, MS, CNRN, ACNP-BC
UC Davis Health
2315 Stockton Boulevard
Sacramento, CA 95817, USA

E-mail address:
cddelemos@ucdavis.edu

REFERENCES

1. Romaine-Davis A. Critical care nursing: a history. Bull Hist Med 1999;73(2):350–1.
2. Williams G, Chaboyer W, Thornsteindóttir R, et al. Worldwide overview of critical care nursing organizations and their activities. Int Nurs Rev 2001;48(4):208–17.
3. Chestnut RM, Temkin N, Carney N, et al. A trial of intracranial-pressure monitoring in traumatic brain injury. N Engl J Med 2012;367(26):2471–81.
4. World Health Organization. Neurologic disorders and public health challenges. 2008. Available at: http://www.who.int/mental_health/neurology/neurodiso/en/. Accessed.

Intensive Care Unit Nursing Priorities in the United States

Sheila A. Alexander, PhD, RN, FCCM

KEYWORDS

- Critical care • Delirium • Mobility • Communication • Palliative care • Tele-ICU
- Care bundles

KEY POINTS

- Nursing research is driving care improvements in the areas of delirium, mobility, communication, palliative care, tele–intensive care unit, and care bundles.
- Delirium prevention and early mobility improve outcomes of ICU patients.
- Effective communication and patient-centered care maximizes patient outcomes and staff, patient, and family satisfaction with care.
- Care bundles provide standard approaches to minimize negative sequelae and maximize outcomes of ICU patients; barriers to bundle implementation can be overcome with focused efforts.
- Nurses have developed methods to decrease Ventilator Associated Pneumonia and Central Line Associate Blood Stream Infections and early identification of Sepsis.

INTRODUCTION/HISTORY/DEFINITIONS/BACKGROUND

The practice of critical care in the United States began long before the first dedicated unit was founded by William Dandy in 1923.[1] Because critically ill patients require increased monitoring and specialized care, they were placed in specific areas or units with equipment and trained personnel able to provide this care; critical care nurses were vital. The practice of critical care nursing was founded on best practice at the time, heavily reliant on expert opinion. The importance of evidence, generated from well-designed research studies, in the management of various health states is now realized as best practice.[2,3] Critical care research from multiple disciplines has informed current best practice.

Nursing practice has evolved based on evidence generated from nurse scientists, and many practices have been abandoned when found to be nonefficacious or

Author funding sources: National Institutes of Health/National Institute of Aging, R21AG.
Acute and Tertiary Care, School of Nursing, Critical Care Medicine, School of Medicine, University of Pittsburgh, 336 Victoria Building, 3500 Victoria Street, Pittsburgh, PA 15261, USA
E-mail address: salexand@pitt.edu

potentially harmful. Nurse scientists conduct research relevant to nursing and patient outcomes and have substantially contributed to evidence-based care in critical care nursing practice.[3] Nurses in the United States conduct research on a variety of critical care topics focused on improving nursing practice and/or patient outcomes. This integrative review reports on the current literature (2015–2019) published by nurse investigators and contributing to the advancement of critical care nursing practice.

Search Terms

A Pubmed search for "Critical Care Nursing Research" limited to humans and English publications from 2015 to 2019 generated 8470 publications; limiting to "US" yielded 249 publications. The search was repeated replacing "Critical Care Nursing Research" with "Nursing Research," yielding 1398 publications; limiting to "US" culled the total number of publications to 296. After removal of duplicate publications, those without a nurse author, those outside the United States, and review articles, there were 59 publications. These publications were categorized into general themes: delirium, early mobility, communication, end-of-life care, tele–intensive care unit (ICU), care bundle implementation, and other research.

Current Evidence: Delirium

Delirium is an acute transient change in cognitive function and consciousness. It is primarily seen in older adults, but in the critical care setting it develops in people of all ages. ICU delirium is associated with poor outcomes, including increased time of mechanical ventilation, increased need for sedative/analgesics, longer ICU and hospital length of stay, increased mortality, and long-term cognitive impairment. Publication of guidelines for management of pain, agitation, and delirium in 2013[4] and the 2018 updated guidelines for management of pain, agitation/sedation, delirium, immobility, and sleep disruption in the ICU[5] have informed nursing research. A substantial amount of nursing research focuses on translation of the ABCDEF (assess, prevent and manage pain; both spontaneous awakening trials and spontaneous breathing trials; choice of analgesia and sedation; delirium assessment, prevention, and management; early mobility and exercise; and family engagement and empowerment) bundle, to improve patient outcomes including delirium, into practice. A bundle is a clear set of guidelines based on current evidence that improve the process of care and that are provided collectively in a consistent manner to improve patient outcomes.[6]

The ABCDEF bundle is an evidence-based guide for the management of ICU patients designed to promote survival and maximize outcomes.[7] The bundle incorporates guidance related to the concepts listed earlier. Pain occurs in up to 50% of ICU patients and requires systematic assessment, prevention, and management in ICU patients.[8] The ABCDEF bundle guidelines recommend frequent assessment, treatment of identified pain, and administration of pain medication before painful procedures.[7] Coordination of daily spontaneous awakening trials and spontaneous breathing trials leads to less time on the ventilator and earlier ICU and hospital discharge.[9] Choice of analgesia and sedation affects patient outcomes; decreased exposure to sedative and analgesic agents, in addition to avoiding benzodiazepines, leads to less delirium, less time on the ventilator, and improved outcomes.[7] Up to 80% of ICU patients develop delirium, which is associated with more time on the ventilator, longer ICU and hospital stays, worse cognitive recovery, and higher mortality.[10] Delirium should be assessed at least every shift, and prevention and management initiatives, such as promoting normal sleep-wake cycles and early mobility, should be initiated to minimize negative sequelae.[7] Early mobility has been shown to decrease delirium and minimize ICU-associated muscle weakness and dysfunction, and should be initiated while in the ICU.[7] Family members are an important part of the critical care team. Engagement of family members as active members of the team during decision making and care planning decreases family anxiety and increases their understanding of care provided but also allows patient preferences to be addressed in care planning.[7] When incorporated as a bundle, these strategies create a culture change and promote optimum patient outcomes. Implementation of the bundle has been shown to decrease delirium incidence and duration,[11,12] mechanical ventilation days, and hospital length of stay[12] in academic medical centers and community hospitals.

Nurse scientists and clinicians have contributed to improvements in delirium recognition and assessment. A multidisciplinary study found subjects with subsyndromal delirium, having only 1 component of delirium, are more likely to be discharged to an institution (rehabilitation facility, long-term acute care facility, nursing home, hospice care, another acute care facility, or other), particularly if subsyndromal delirium lasts for 5 days.[13] Additional research has focused on defining distinct delirium phenotypes, defined as clinical risk factors, and their relationship to long-term cognitive impairment. One study identified 5 delirium phenotypes: hypoxic, septic, sedative, metabolic, and unclassified. After controlling for relevant variables, longer duration of hypoxic, septic, sedative, and unclassified delirium phenotypes, but not metabolic delirium phenotype, were associated with poorer cognition.[14]

Delirium is a multifactorial condition without an identified cause. Preexisting cognitive impairment; mechanical ventilation; untreated pain; use of sedatives, analgesics, and other psychoactive drugs; immobilization; severity of injury/illness; common comorbidities; sepsis; and sleep deprivation are risk factors that contribute to the development of delirium.[7] Nursing interventions can be applied to minimize delirium risk and often thwart its development altogether. Frequent assessment identifies delirium as soon as it develops and can prompt treatments to decrease delirium duration.[7] Review of medications to avoid polypharmacy and avoidance of deliriogenic medications is an important nursing intervention to prevent or minimize the effects of delirium.[15] Nurses also promote and organize early mobility when it is safe and provide interventions to promote sleep and maintenance of a normal circadian rhythm to prevent delirium.[5,7]

Current Evidence: Early Mobility

Early mobility in ICU patients improves patient outcomes. Nurse-led and team mobilization protocols have been shown to increase the likelihood of mobility. Consideration of mobilization of ICU patients should begin on admission. Passive range of motion and turning should be used until more advanced mobilization can occur. As patients become more stable, semi-Fowler position, standing and pivoting to a chair, and ultimately ambulation can occur with assistance and coordination by the nurse. When a patient is able to successfully sit, ambulation may occur.[16] Patients need to be hemodynamically stable for mobilization, and without certain contraindications (eg, deep vein thrombosis). Sedative use should also be considered because it is important for patients to be able to interact with clinicians and follow directions during mobilization. Respiratory needs increase during mobilization and it is often necessary to increase respiratory support to meet those needs during mobilization. Early mobility requires substantial resources. The nurse should evaluate which intravenous fluids can be halted and which need to be continued and monitored throughout the mobility experience. Portable telemetry is used to monitor the patient. A respiratory therapist is needed to manage a portable ventilator (or manual resuscitation bag) for respiration and ventilation. Catheters and drainage tubes must be secured before mobilization. During the mobilization, the nurse monitors vital signs for stability and additional personnel assist the patient with mobilization.[17] There are differences in mobility practices by institution,[16] and research designed to facilitate mobility in all units is ongoing. Benefits of early mobility include a reduction in hospital-acquired pressure ulcer incidence. Azuh and colleagues[18] (2016) developed a mobility team including a new patient mobility assistant. The team then implemented a protocol to evaluate ICU patients for mobility and baseline function, develop and implement an individual mobility plan, and evaluate function and modify the plan accordingly during the patients' ICU stays. They reported a decrease in acquired pressure ulcer rate, 1-day decrease in ICU length of stay, and a decrease in hospital readmission after discharge. Although they showed the positive benefits of early mobilization of ICU patients, they also showed that, with proper training, the unlicensed patient mobility assistant was able to safely facilitate early mobilization at less cost in clinician time.[18]

Although early mobility is associated with improved outcome after ICU admission, optimal administration is under investigation. A nurse-led mobility protocol was initiated in 4 ICUs. Patients requiring mechanical ventilation for more than 48 hours were randomized to once-daily or twice-daily early therapeutic mobilization. Twice-daily mobilization was associated with shorter ICU length of stay. Out-of-bed mobility was associated with increased muscle strength at ICU discharge and decreased delirium.[19] In a recent study of use of a mobility team, patients in the early mobility group had fewer falls, ventilator-associated events, pressure ulcers, catheter-associated urinary tract infections, and delirium days, and lower sedation needs and costs. In addition, the early mobility group had higher functional independence and no adverse events.[20]

Krupp and colleagues[21] (2019) sought to identify barriers to widespread implementation of early mobility through semistructured interviews. Nurses reported that the purpose of mobility included preventing complications, meeting unit standards, and assisting patients in achieving individual goals. They gathered relevant information from verbal and written communication, baseline patient testing, watching, and knowing the patient. Establishing and activating the plan barriers included being the first to mobilize the patient, determining patient acuity and matching goals, determining patient response to mobilization, and coordinating the patient and resources. Additional barriers included resource use, unit activity, patient availability, and variation in individual nurse practice of mobility.[21] A survey of critical care professionals from a research-intensive unit found few reported barriers, particularly from those clinicians with greater than 10 years' experience. When analyzing perceived barriers by years of experience, each year of experience was associated with decreased reported barriers up to 10 years. This finding suggests that, as providers practice mobilizing patients, skillset and confidence improve. Not surprisingly, nurses reported the highest level of barriers, whereas attending physicians reported the lowest. Although the investigators did not report granular data on specific barriers to mobility identified by each group, nurses identified lower knowledge barriers compared with physicians and advanced practice providers. This finding suggests that the nurses responding to this survey perceive barriers related to practical application of early mobility rather than a lack of knowledge of how to mobilize patients or the benefits of early mobility.[22] This body of work highlights the significant barriers to early mobilization at the individual nurse, patient, unit, and institutional level. Education about the benefits of mobility, appropriate mobility for individual ICU patients based on current physiologic state, and safe procedures for mobility is required for all ICU providers. In addition, available resources and staff to safely mobilize patients, consistent goals for mobilizing every patient every day at an appropriate level, and adequate staffing to ensure that daily mobilization can occur on a busy unit are important concepts for successful implementation of a mobility protocol in the ICU.

Current Evidence: Communication

During ICU admission, patients are often intubated and mechanically ventilated, which impairs communication and care. Options to facilitate communication with these ICU patients are few; however, the Study of Patient-Nurse Effectiveness with Assisted Communication Strategies (SPEACS) program is an excellent multiarmed program to improve communication. It incorporates nurse education on alternative communication devices and speech language pathologist consultation.[23] The SPEACS program increases nurses' knowledge, satisfaction, and comfort when communicating with intubated, mechanically ventilated patients. It did not change physical restraint use, use of heavy sedation, pain score documentation, pressure ulcer presence, coma-free days, ventilator-free days, ICU or hospital length of stay, or median cost.[24]

Although the SPEACS program improves communication for patients, additional work is designed to improve clinicians' communication with one another. Gunter and colleagues[25] (2019) developed a tool to facilitate multidisciplinary communication during rounds. The tool provides a platform for consistently presenting concise, accurate, and relevant patient information. The tool has been positively received by the multidisciplinary team and its use has been expanded to include nursing handoffs.[25]

Because nursing research informs how US clinicians communicate with one another and their patients, there is also evidence it is informing communication with patients' family members. A study recorded conversations between clinicians and surrogate decision makers about patient care goals and analyzed them for inclusion of patient treatment preferences and values. Patient preferences and values were discussed in 68.4% of these conversations, with discussion of direct application to goals of care occurring in 44.3%. Despite this, surrogates provided substitute judgment in 13.5% and clinicians made recommendations based on patient preferences and values in only 8.2% of conversations. This work highlights the need for improved communication but also improvements in clinician application of patient preferences and values to care.[26] Communication and collaboration of team members is important for family members of ICU patients. When surveyed, family caregivers valued interprofessional communication within the team, patient/family-centered care, roles and responsibilities, and values and ethics within team members. Teamwork scores positively correlate with satisfaction with care in the ICU.[27]

Current Evidence: Family Engagement

From surrogate decision making to participation in direct care, nurses are driving improvements in the ICU experience based on family engagement. In a large, multicenter, multidisciplinary study, clinician support and guidance for improved family engagement was provided via monthly team calls, quarterly webinars, newsletters, an online community, and team reporting assignments. Family members reported improved satisfaction overall and specifically in decision making and quality of care. Clinicians reported improved family involvement but also barriers, including lack of buy-in and ability to effect change in their environments, workload associated with implementation, and financial challenges.[28]

A qualitative study explored practices to increase family engagement in care. Not all family members can or should participate in care of ICU patients. Individual assessment of willingness and ability must be considered for each task, and individual nurses have different opinions leading to variable practice within an individual unit. End-of-life care was considered an acceptable place for families to participate in care by all respondents.[29]

Family engagement is heavily influenced by visiting hours. Open visiting hours, when visitors are welcome at any time, is of benefit to both families and patients. Because there are inconsistent practices in ICUs within an institution as well as across multiple institutions around the country, Suba and colleagues[30] explored the influence of unit-based clinical nurse specialist but found no differences. A family member survey study conducted in a unit with open visitation found family needs were met, particularly related to receiving patient status updates, visitation, having hope supported, connecting with the physician daily, and assurance regarding receipt of best care. Although the study findings are limited, the investigators concluded that the open visitation hours and a private suite for family members contributed to the positive results.[31]

The coronavirus disease 2019 (COVID-19) pandemic introduced significant challenges to family engagement because of restrictions placed on visitors of patients in hospitals and ICUs. There is institutional variability in visitation policies of ICU patients. Many facilities banned all visitors, some restricted all visitors but provided some exceptions, and some restricted visitors to 1 per patient.[32] It is difficult to engage families, and these practices have created significant distress for patients, family members, and clinicians. Clinicians have shifted to telephone calls as the primary means of communication with family members, with some using video conferencing. Many facilities instituted video communication for patient-family communications, although this was sometimes impaired by lack of resources.[32] Although the COVID-19 pandemic is ongoing, early reports have shown that delirium rates are high in these patients,[33] which may be exacerbated by visitor limitations. Patients with COVID-19 also report feeling socially isolated, which contributes to stress, anxiety, and depression that challenges recovery in the ICU and beyond.[34] Family members are unable to participate as care partners with such limited communication and this is likely to contribute to their risk of anxiety and depression. The altered communication mechanisms are also proposed to contribute to moral distress in caregivers.[35] As the COVID-19 pandemic continues, health care providers must balance the public health initiatives with individual needs to create individual visitation and communication plans that serve the needs of each patient-family unit.

Current Evidence: End-of-Life Care

Although advances in critical care practice have improved survival rates, mortality is high. ICU patients are extremely sick and often have multiple comorbidities contributing to the poor outcomes. Death is a common outcome for ICU patients; nurse scientists are exploring end-of-life care and driving the movement for peaceful and painless death.

A large study from the ICU Liberation Collaborative described the processes, structures, and variability provided at the end of life in ICUs in the United States. Most facilities (78%) had open visitation during end-of-life care. At the individual patient level, about 40% had advanced directives, 10.5% had cardiopulmonary resuscitation in the hour before death, 65% were extubated before death, 60% were delirium free 24 hours before death, 75% were pain free 24 hours before death, and 88% had family present at death. Variability in end-of-life care is influenced by advanced practice providers, protocol presence/adherence, unit culture, and ethical climate.[36] The presence of advanced directives before admission in older adults is low (42%) but an important component for providing appropriate end-of-life care, suggesting a need for education of the public.[37] A report on clinician experiences from the 3 Wishes Project, which focuses on implementing palliative care measures based on patient wishes, found the initiative enhanced palliative care practice and positively influenced clinicians and patient families.[38] Palliative care–specialized advanced practice nurses reduced hospital costs per patient in 1 institution but not another.[39] A survey of 1173 nurses in the Seattle/Tacoma Washington area found that nurses perceived a higher-quality death when physician-family communication was strong and particularly when physicians supported family decision making. Of interest, the nurses concern for the patient or family was associated with a lower-quality death. These results suggest areas for improvement in promoting a high-quality death in the ICU.[40]

Nurses are concerned about end-of-life care in ICU patients, and recent evidence shows that there are gaps in its efficacy and areas for improvement. Nurses reported there were consistent symptoms at the end of life (eg, breathing, edema, limb control loss), and treatment was often only partially effective, contributing to increased suffering and loss of dignity for the patient.[41] In a large survey of nurses, ensuring a good death, improved communication between physicians and family members, improved staffing ratios (nurses and support staff), improved recognition and avoidance of futile care, increasing education, and adhering to patient wishes were all important but inconsistent practices when providing end-of-life care. These suggestions are very similar to results from a survey conducted 17 years ago; there is a consistent need for improvement.[42]

Dionne-Odom and colleagues[43] have developed a framework for end-of-life decision making by surrogates in the ICU. They found gist impressions (defined as salient impressions emerging from family meetings, interactions with health care providers, and visual images of their loved ones in the ICU), distressing emotions, and moral intuitions were impactful factors on acceptability of the patients' medical care or condition.[43]

Bereavement care for family members of patients who die in the ICU must be approached with consideration of the individual. Family members positively viewed bereavement resources and brochures, but there was variability in specific components preferred. Unit-based counseling services were helpful in processing grief. The memory box and sympathy card received mixed reviews. Most families would not have attended a memorial service and found the follow-up telephone call unnecessary.[44] Bereavement needs of ICU patient families vary and warrant an individual approach.

Health care providers are also concerned about the lack of bereavement care offered. Nurse managers reported that most institutions did not offer follow-up bereavement services for family members. Bereavement care that was offered was limited and primarily in the form of brochures and condolence cards. Bereavement services were available at a much higher rate in institutions with palliative care services. Reported barriers to offering bereavement services included lack of education, financial constraints, knowledge gaps, lack of expertise, and time.[45]

As part of ICU care, goals-of-care discussions are important and necessary, often leading to palliative care and/or end-of-life care. Goals-of-care discussions should occur early in the ICU stay and be multidisciplinary, including all clinicians involved in care and the family. Physicians often present the medical data about the case, discuss care options, and provide prognostic information. Nurses can contribute to discussion related to appropriateness of the goals of care and, if needed, practical aspects of initiating palliative care.[46] Because ICU patients are often not able to speak for themselves, nurses must advocate for the patients. Learning about the patients' life stories and identifying the patients' goals and preferences may occur through interaction with the patients or the families during routine care or a formal goals-of-care discussion. At all times the nurses must advocate for the patients, making sure their goals and preferences are incorporated into the plan. ICU nurses also assess and manage common end-of-life issues, including pain, agitation, and dyspnea.

Assessment findings should be shared with the team to inform goals of care before and during end of life. Nurses also serve as a source of knowledge and support for families during and after goals-of-care discussions.[47]

Current Evidence: Tele–Intensive Care Unit

Use of tele-ICU provides an opportunity for increased services by specialists better meeting the needs of patients and supporting clinicians. Tele-ICU uses an off-site command center to electronically connect clinicians at an area of need with expert clinicians. Tele-ICU decreases mortality, especially in high-volume urban hospitals,[48] and has positive influences on access to care and finances.[49] In a recent survey of bedside nurses to identify perceptions of tele-ICU, with a follow-up Delphi approach to set nursing priorities for tele-ICU, nurses positively viewed tele-ICU services. Tele-ICU improved collaboration, communication, job performance, and care quality. Priority areas of care facilitated by tele-ICU identified were critical thinking skills, intensive care experience, communication, mutual respect, and management of emergency patient care.[50] Tele-ICU services also decreased failure to rescue by focusing on support and clinical coordination interventions.[51]

In an effort to decrease transmission of the novel coronavirus, severe acute respiratory syndrome coronavirus-2 (SARS-Cov-2), telehealth services have been used at a rapidly increasing rate. Because ICUs were in very high demand, many nurses and other health care providers who normally do not work in the ICU were assigned to care for patients requiring ICU care. Many facilities, including Atrium Health, relied on tele-ICU services to ensure care that was safe for both patients and providers. Nurses, physicians, and other providers used tele-ICU technology to train staff on high-risk procedures and donning/doffing personal protective equipment, consult on critical care provision, perform virtual assessments of patients in isolation, communicate with nurses inside the rooms, and deliver supplies needed to limit both providers in the room but also frequency of entering/leaving the room.[52]

Current Evidence: Care Bundle Implementation

Care in the ICU is complex. Several care bundles, or protocols focused on common problems for ICU patients, have been developed. Implementation of bundles is challenging in many ICUs but there are strategies to improve implementation. The ABCDE (2011) and ABCDEF (2017) bundles, developed by multidisciplinary teams, have been commonly used as a protocol for ICU care.[5,53–55] The ICU Liberation Collaborative found that in academic, community, and federal ICUs, implementation of the ABCDEF bundle was feasible and meaningfully improved patient outcomes.[56] Others have reported similar improvement in patient outcomes after bundle implementation,[57,58] including in long-term acute care settings.[59]

Successful implementation of the ABCDEF bundle depends on inclusion of multiple team members, including nurses, physicians, and nursing assistants.[60] A multidisciplinary survey of ICU providers found that implementation was impaired by barriers including workload burden, complexity of the bundle, confidence in the implementation, safety issues, and strength of evidence for bundle components.[61] Unpredictable team member behavior, meaning that members did not always know that another team member would behave in a certain way and apply each aspect of the bundle for a given patient, is also a barrier to bundle implementation.[62] There are many facilitators of bundle adoption: protocol attributes, provider role clarity, task autonomy, provider education and understanding of the protocol, coordination of care, teamwork, and peer advocates were associated with ease of protocol use and positive provider attitude about the bundle.[63]

Detection and Early Management of Infectious Processes: Sepsis, Central Line–Associated Blood Stream Infections and Ventilator-Associated Pneumonia

Sepsis and infection control are consistent topics in the medical and nursing research literature. Sepsis is common in ICU patients, and a multidisciplinary, international collaborative group generated the "Surviving Sepsis Campaign: International Guidelines for Management of Sepsis and Septic Shock" in 2016.[64] Although review of nursing implications for that entire document is beyond the scope of this article, aspects with particular relevance for nurses have been published and include several key nursing roles. Monitoring of vital signs, sepsis screening, and activation of the sepsis team (if available) or initiation of sepsis care protocols are nursing roles important for sepsis screening. Sepsis treatment measures performed by nurses include obtaining blood cultures before antibiotic administration, administering antibiotics, and fluid resuscitation. Ongoing monitoring of vital signs, laboratory values, signs of altered perfusion, and administering medication and other interventions as ordered promote maximum recovery. Nurses should maintain familiarity with the current sepsis guidelines and disseminate relevant information from these guidelines to the care team, including clinicians in the ICU, emergency department, and ward staff. In addition to educating others about the sepsis management guidelines, nurses should also target sepsis in quality-improvement initiatives. In addition, nurses should make infection control measures a priority in the ICU.[65]

Infection control is a priority for ICU nurses outside of its relevance to sepsis. Central line–associated blood stream infection (CLABSI) is a blood stream infection developing within 48 hours of central line insertion, confirmed by a laboratory but not associated with another infectious site. Prevention of these infections is key to improving patient outcomes and primarily relies on nursing care. There are many published care bundles addressing CLABSI prevention. Most commonly these include a combination of (1) hand hygiene before insertion, (2) maximal barrier precautions, (3) chlorhexidine skin preparation before catheter insertion and during maintenance, (4) central line placement into the subclavian vein or internal jugular vein rather than the femoral vein, and (5) daily review of line necessity with removal as early as possible.[66] Nursing monitoring of sterility during central line placement, replacement of central lines with peripheral intravenous catheters, regular dressing changes to maintain a clean and dry dressing over the insertion site, use of chlorhexidine gluconate Tegaderm dressings, and use of proper line access when needed decrease CLABSI incidence to near zero.[67] Additional work has shown that staff education and commitment to practicing in ways that reduce CLABSI are effective in decreasing CLABSI rates.[68] There is variability in incorporation of and adherence to these bundles. One survey found that, in institutions with bundle policies in place, only 69% reported greater than or equal to 85% compliance with at least 1 element. Having a policy in place did not associate with infection rates, but compliance with 1 or more elements decreased infection rates, with larger reduction seen with more element compliance.[66]

Ventilator-associated pneumonia (VAP) is a common nosocomial infection in the United States with an incidence of 2 to 16 per 1000 ventilator days.[69] Prevention methods for VAP begin with minimizing intubation when possible, minimizing sedation and conducting spontaneous awakening trials daily, early mobilization, changing ventilator circuit tubing, oral care with chlorhexidine, subglottal secretion drainage, in some instances administration of prophylactic probiotics, and maintaining the head of the bed at a 30° to 45° angle.[70]

Table 1
Other research

Topic	Purpose/Hypotheses	Findings	Reference
Alarm fatigue	To examine the effectiveness and acceptance of physiologic monitor software to support customization of alarms	Use of alarm customization software was associated with increased use of alarms and decreased nuisance alarms. Nurses reported less time spent on nonactionable alarms, less disturbance to workflow, and fewer instances where there was not a response to an important alarm	Ruppel et al,[71] 2018
Fatigue	To describe levels of fatigue and explore clinical factors that might contribute to fatigue in critically ill patients receiving mechanical ventilation	Baseline mean fatigue ratings were high (69 out of 100 mm on a visual analog scale). Illness severity and more frequent sedative administration were related to higher fatigue ratings in these mechanically ventilated patients	Chlan and Savik,[72] 2015
Hemorrhage	To determine the rate of rectal tube hemorrhage among patients in a transplant ICU	Incidence rate of rectal tube associated hemorrhage was 3%	Glass et al,[73] 2018
Infection	To examine the relationship between nursing job satisfaction and health care–associated infections in adult critical care	Nurses' satisfaction with organizational policies and favorable perception of task requirements were associated with fewer health care–associated infections. Nurses' perception of pay, autonomy, and interactions were associated with increased health care–associated infections. Units with a higher proportion of critical care registered nurses and certified nurses had lower rates of health care–associated infections	Boev et al,[74] 2015
Infection	To explore the impact of legislation and mandatory reporting on central-line–associated blood stream infection rates and reporting	The number of reported central-line–associated blood stream infections decreased over time, although the sample size is too small to draw conclusions regarding the impact of legislation	Woodward et al,[75] 2018
Infection	To examine the variability in catheter-associated asymptomatic bacteriuria-free outcomes of individual nurses	Catheter-associated asymptomatic bacteriuria-free rates of individual nurses varied between 94 and 100 per 100 shifts	Yakusheva et al,[76] 2019

Maximize physical outcomes	To compare standardized rehabilitation therapy with usual ICU care in acute respiratory failure	Standardized rehabilitation therapy did not decrease hospital or ICU length of stay, days of mechanical ventilation. At 6 mo after discharge, the standardized rehabilitation therapy group had higher physical and functional performance scores compared with the usual ICU care group	Morris et al,[77] 2016
Mortality prediction	To examine the association between BAC at hospital admission and risk of 30-d mortality in critically ill patients	A positive blood alcohol level on admission is associated with decreased mortality	Stehman et al,[78] 2015
Mortality prediction	To determine whether a low Braden skin score predicts lower survival in cardiac ICU patients after adjustment for illness severity and comorbidities	Admission Braden skin score inversely associated with hospital mortality and postdischarge mortality even after controlling for relevant variables	Jentzer et al,[79] 2019
Pain	The investigators hypothesize that there is inadequate pain control and introduction of the critical care pain observation tool could improve it	Adequacy of pain control was 78%, higher than the 71% reported in the literature; pain control increased to 99% with introduction of the critical care pain observation tool	D'Andrea et al,[80] 2017
Pressure ulcer	To identify factors associated with pressure ulcer development in a medical ICU	The presence of hemodynamic support with vasopressor agents and increased length of stay were associated with pressure ulcer development. There was no association between pressure ulcer development and age, sex, comorbidities (number), primary diagnosis, or mortality	Smit et al,[81] 2016
Restraint reduction	To decrease use of restraints in a medical-surgical ICU and to determine whether a decision support tool is useful in helping bedside nurses determine whether or not to restrain a patient	Restraint use decreased by 32%, with an increase in adverse events, after implementation of the decision-making support tool	Hevener et al,[82] 2019
Sleep	To test the impact of an ICU sleep promotion protocol on overnight in-room disturbance	During a rest time block (00:00–04:00) individuals in the sleep promotion protocol had 32% fewer room entries and 9.1% fewer minutes of in-room activity	Knauert et al,[83] 2019

(continued on next page)

Table 1
(continued)

Topic	Purpose/Hypotheses	Findings	Reference
Sleep	To explore the perceptions and beliefs of staff, patients, and surrogates regarding the environmental and nonenvironmental factors in the medical ICU that affect patients' sleep	This qualitative study found 4 themes: overnight unit environment does affect sleep, nonenvironmental factors also affect sleep, perceptions of sleep quality in the ICU are variable, and respondents had suggestions to improve sleep	Ding et al,[84] 2017

Research on topics not covered in depth in the article are listed. They are organized by major topic areas. The overall purpose, goal, aims and/or hypotheses, major findings, and reference list number are provided.
Abbreviation: BAC, Blood Alcohol Concentration.

Current Evidence: Other Research

Evidence supporting critical care practice is growing exponentially. This large body of work includes additional research focused on many areas, as well as work not included in this review because it was focused on a very specific population or had minimal direct clinical application. **Table 1** reports the general purpose and findings of additional studies. These projects focus on symptom and complication management, nursing practice challenges, and patient outcomes.

DISCUSSION

US critical care nursing has come a long way from the first ICUs where care was solely driven by physician preference. Nurse scientists continue to build the evidence base and translate that evidence into clinical practice. The role of the doctor of nursing practice has facilitated the translation of research findings into the clinical realm and generated new evidence supporting effective and practical approaches to that translation. Nurses are contributing to the advancement of nursing science in a substantial way, developing evidence that drives their practice.[85] Nursing research allows nurses to own their science, driving the development of the profession, and be held accountable for its advancement and translation.

The research reviewed here shows how nurses are contributing to improved patient outcomes through increased recognition and care for patients with ICU delirium, increased safe delivery of early mobility, improving communication with their patients and their peers, supporting one another through tele-ICU provision, and promoting standardization of care through bundle implementation.

There is a wealth of research from all disciplines focused on ICU delirium, from recognition to treatment and outcomes. Most medication trials have not shown efficacy,[4,5,86,87] although sedation/analgesic dose should be minimized.[4,5,8,54] Environmental modification may decrease delirium incidence and duration.[7,12] Early mobility decreases delirium and has many other benefits for maximizing patient outcomes.[7,18,20,88] There are practical challenges to its application, but the nursing research presented here is addressing this need.[18–20,88] Improving communication with ICU patients is primarily a nursing endeavor, whereas communication with other health care professionals and family members is a multidisciplinary effort showing that improved communication skills are necessary for ICU clinicians.[24–26,89,90] End-of-life care and bundle implementation are primarily driven by nurses either independently or within teams. Tele-ICU is used by multiple clinicians to improve clinician performance and patient outcomes.[91] Infection control protocols have been developed and are being implemented with significant contributions from nurses, leading to lower rates of CLABSI and VAP.[64–68] Nursing research is improving nursing care in the ICU but also informing the practice of other disciplines, ultimately leading to better outcomes for patients and their families.

SUMMARY

Advancements in nursing science on the topics of delirium, early mobility, communication, end-of-life care, tele-ICU, and bundle implementation are highlighted here. Contributions to the literature on ICU delirium include improvements to assessment and prevention with a focus on different presentations. Nurses are driving the research on early mobility, reporting on timing, dose, and frequency as well as promoting consistent provision of this treatment. Evidence is growing on tools and approaches to communication with ICU patients but also best practices for communication with family members and other health care providers. Nurses are leading the movement for palliative care in the ICU, with a focus on improving both quantity and quality of this service. Tele-ICU is a new approach where nurses are finding a niche to support to one another while improving patient outcomes. Standardized protocols have been in existence for many years, but, with current trends for bundling care for maximum patient benefit, nurses are leading the way for proper and practical translation of these bundles into use in the ICU. Protocols and bundles promoting best practices in infection control are decreasing the frequency of nosocomial infections and improving outcomes for all ICU patients

CLINICS CARE POINTS

Delirium
- Incorporate delirium assessment, prevention, and treatment into routine care; consider unit-level initiation of the ABCDEF bundle to maximize patient outcomes.
- Monitor patients for subsyndromal delirium, and specific phenotype, treating appropriately to maximize outcomes.

Early mobility
- Mobilize patients at the appropriate level throughout the ICU stay.
- Create a mobility team to focus on safe, practical, and efficacious mobility practices.
- Promote a culture change that encourages daily mobility of every patient.

Communication
- Use every tool available to communicate with patients; consider the SPEACS program.
- Maintain collaborative communication styles with colleagues from all professions.
- Communicate frequently about goals and status with patients and their families.

Family engagement
- Family involvement in care requires careful assessment of willingness and ability.
- Encourage visitation of family members and adapt to video conferencing when in-person visitation must be limited.
- There are numerous barriers to full family engagement. Promote an environment that supports family members and their engagement, flexible visiting hours, frequent communication with family members, and honesty and reassurance in communication.

End-of-life care
- Communication is key.
- Initiate goals-of-care discussion early.
- Consider patient preferences and values, advocate for the patient.
- Provide care and alleviate symptoms in a way that maintains dignity.
- Incorporate providers with palliative care expertise when possible.
- Provide support to family members during and after decision making.

Tele-ICU
- Sharing expertise, or receiving guidance based on expertise, improves patient outcomes.
- Use tele-ICU approaches to assist other nurses with expertise outside the ICU currently working in ICU environments.

Bundle implementation

- Bundle protocols provide standardized care, improving patient outcomes.
- Engage all disciplines, through education and defining specific roles, when implementing.
- Provide education, direction, and support to new or less experienced clinicians when implementing bundles.

Detection and early management of infectious processes

- Incorporate bundle protocols in standardized care, improving patient outcomes for sepsis, CLABSI, and VAP.
- Maintain current knowledge of best practices in the prevention, monitoring, and treatment of sepsis, CLABSI, and VAP.
- Monitor patients for signs and symptoms of infectious processes, promptly report significant findings.
- Incorporate best-practice infection prevention into clinical practice; promote unit-level protocols and monitoring for infectious processes.

DISCLOSURE

The author has nothing to disclose.

REFERENCES

1. Vincent JL. Critical care- where we have been and where we are going. Crit Care 2013;17(S2). https://doi.org/10.1186/cc11500.
2. Youngblut JM, Brooten D. Evidence-based nursing practice: why is it important? AACN Clin Issues 2001;12(4):468–76.
3. Stevens K. The impact of evidence-based practice in nursing and the next big idea. Online J Issues Nurs 2013;18(2). https://doi.org/10.3912/OJIN.Vol18No02Man04. manuscript 4.
4. Barr J, Fraser GL, Puntillo K, et al. Clinical practice guidelines for the management of pain, agitation, and delirium in adult patients in the intensive care unit. Crit Care Med 2013;41(1):263–306.
5. Devlin JW, Skrobik Y, Gelinas C, et al. Clinical practice guidelines for the management of pain, agitation/sedation, delirium, immobility, and sleep disruptions in adult patients in the ICU. Crit Care Med 2018;46(9):e825–73.
6. Institute for Healthcare Improvement. Bundles: evidence based care bundles. Institute for healthcare improvement website. Available at: http://www.ihi.org/Topics/Bundles/Pages/default.aspx. Accessed October 3, 2020.
7. Marra A, Ely EW, Pandharipande PP, et al. The ABCDEF bundle in critical care. Crit Care Clin 2017;33(2):225–43.
8. Payen JF, Chanques G, Mantz J, et al. Current practices in sedation and analgesia for mechanically ventilated critically ill patients: a prospective multicenter patient-based study. Anesthesiology 2007;106(4):687–95.
9. Girard TD, Kress JP, Fuchs BD, et al. Efficacy and safety of a paired sedation and ventilator weaning protocol for mechanically ventilated patients in intensive care (Awakening and breathing controlled trial): a randomised controlled trial. Lancet 2008;371(9607):126–34.
10. Salluh JI, Wang H, Schneider EB, et al. Outcome of delirium in critically ill patients: systematic review and meta-analysis. BMJ 2015;350:h2538.

11. Bounds M, Kram S, Gabel Speroni K, et al. Effect of ABCDE bundle implementation on prevalence of delirium in intensive care unit patients. Am J Crit Care 2016;25(6):535–44.

12. Kram SL, DiBartolo MC, Hinderer K, et al. Implementation of the ABCDE bundle to improve patient outcomes in the intensive care unit in a rural community hospital. Dimens Crit Care Nurs 2015;34(5):250–8.

13. Brummel NE, Boehm LM, Girard TD, et al. Subsyndromal delirium and institutionalization among patients with critical illness. Am J Crit Care 2017;26(6):447–55.

14. Girard TD, Thompson JL, Pandharipande PP, et al. Clinical phenotypes of delirium during critical illness and severity of subsequent long-term cognitive impairment: a prospective cohort study. Lancet Respir Med 2018;6(3):213–22.

15. Damluji AA, Forman DE, van Diepen S, et al. American heart association council on clinical cardiology and council on cardiovascular and stroke nursing. older adults in the cardiac intensive care unit: factoring geriatric syndromes in the management, prognosis, and process of care: a scientific statement from the American heart association. Circulation 2020;141(2):e6–32.

16. Stolldorf DP, Dietrich MS, Chidume T, et al. Nurse-initiated mobilization practices in 2 community intensive care units: a pilot study. Dimens Crit Care Nurs 2018;37(6):318–23.

17. Perme C, Chandrashekhar R. Early mobility and walking program for patients in the intensive care units: creating a standard of care. Am J Crit Care 2009;18(3):212–21.

18. Azuh O, Gammon H, Burmeister C, et al. Benefits of early active mobility in the medical intensive care unit: a pilot study. Am J Med 2016;129(8):866–71.

19. Winkelman C, Satter A, Momatz H, et al. Dose of early therapeutic mobility: does frequency or intensity matter? Biol Res Nurs 2018;20(5):522–30.

20. Fraser D, Spiva L, Forman W, et al. Original research: implementation of an early mobility program in an ICU. Am J Nurs 2015;115(12):49–58.

21. Krupp AE, Ehlenbach WJ, King B. Factors nurses in the intensive care unit consider when making decisions about patient mobility. Am J Crit Care 2019;28(4):281–9.

22. Goodson CM, Aronson Friedman L, Mantheiy E, et al. Perceived barriers to mobility in a medical ICU: the patient mobilization attitudes & beliefs survey for the ICU. J Intensive Care Med 2018;35(10):1026–31.

23. Happ MB, Garrett KL, Tate JA, et al. Effect of a multi-level intervention on nurse-patient communication in the intensive care unit: results of the SPEACS trial. Heart Lung 2014;43(2):89–98.

24. Happ MB, Sereika S, Houze MP, et al. Quality of care and resource use among mechanically ventilated patients before and after an intervention to assist nurse-nonvocal patient communication. Heart Lung 2015;44(5):408–15.e2.

25. Gunter EP, Viswanathan M, Stutzman SE, et al. Development and testing of an electronic multidisciplinary rounding tool. AACN Adv Crit Care 2019;30(3):222–9.

26. Scheunemann LP, Ernecoff NC, Buddadhumaruk P, et al. Clinician-family communication about patients' values and preferences in intensive care units. JAMA Intern Med 2019;179(5):676–84.

27. Chen DW, Gerolamo AM, Harmon E, et al. Interprofessional collaborative practice in the medical intensive care unit: a survey of caregivers perspectives. J Gen Intern Med 2018;33(10):1708–13.

28. Kleinpell R, Zimmerman J, Vermoch KL, et al. Promoting family engagement in the ICU: experience from a national collaborative of 63 ICUs. Crit Care Med 2019;47(12):1692–8.

29. Hetland B, McAndrew N, Perazzo J, et al. A qualitative study of factors that influence active family involvement with patient care in the ICU: survey of critical care nurses. Intensive Crit Care Nurs 2018;44:67–75.

30. Suba S, Donesky D, Scruth EA, et al. Association between clinical nurse specialist's presence and open visitation in US intensive care units. Clin Nurse Spec 2017;31(1):30–5.

31. Jacob M, Horton C, Rance-Ashley S, et al. Needs of patients' family members in an intensive care unit with continuous visitation. Am J Crit Care 2016;25(2): 118–25.

32. Valley TS, Schutz A, Nagle MT, et al. Changes to visitation policies and communication practices in Michigan ICUs during the COVID-19 pandemic. Am J Respir Crit Care Med 2020;202(6):883–5.

33. Kotfis K, Williams Roberson S, Wilson JE, et al. COVID-19: ICU delirium management during SARS-CoV-2 pandemic. Crit Care 2020;24(1):176.

34. Life Lines Team comprising. Restricted family visiting in intensive care during COVID-19. Intensive Crit Care Nurs 2020;60:102896.

35. Greenberg N, Docherty M, Gnanapragasam S, et al. Managing mental health challenges faced by healthcare workers during covid-19 pandemic. BMJ 2020; 368:m1211.

36. Kruser JM, Aaby DA, Stevenson DG, et al. Assessment of variability in end-of-life care delivery in intensive care units in the United States. JAMA Netw Open 2019; 2(12):e1917344.

37. Gamertsfelder EM, Seaman JB, Tate J, et al. Prevalence of advance directives among older adults admitted to intensive care units and requiring mechanical ventilation. J Gerontol Nurs 2016;42(4):34–41.

38. Neville TH, Agarwal N, Swinton M, et al. Improving end-of-life care in the intensive care unit: clinicians' experiences with the 3 wishes project. J Palliat Med 2019; 22(12):1561–7.

39. O'Mahony S, Johnson TJ, Amer S, et al. Integration of palliative care advanced practice nurses into intensive care unit teams. Am J Hosp Palliat Care 2017; 34(4):330–4.

40. Ramos KJ, Downey L, Nielsen EL, et al. Using nurse ratings of physician communication in the ICU to identify potential targets for interventions to improve end-of-life care. J Palliat Med 2016;19(3):292–9.

41. Su A, Lief L, Berlin D, et al. Beyond pain: nurses' assessment of patient suffering, dignity, and dying in the intensive care unit. J Pain Symptom Manage 2018;55(6): 1591–8.e1.

42. Beckstrand RL, Hadley KH, Luthy KE, et al. Critical care nurses' suggestions to improve end-of-life care obstacles: minimal change over 17 years. Crit Care Nurse 2017;36(4):264–70.

43. Dionne-Odom JN, Willis DG, Bakitas M, et al. Conceptualizing surrogate decision making at end of life in the intensive care unit using cognitive task analysis. Nurs Outlook 2015;63(3):331–40.

44. Erikson A, Puntillo K, McAdam J. Family members' opinions about bereavement care after cardiac intensive care unit patients' deaths. Nurs Crit Care 2019;24(4): 209–21.

45. McAdam JL, Erikson A. Bereavement services offered in adult intensive care units in the United States. Am J Crit Care 2016;25(2):110–7.

46. Frontera JA, Curtis JR, Nelson JE, et al. Integrating palliative care into the care of neurocritically Ill patients: a report from the improving palliative care in the ICU

project advisory board and the center to advance palliative care. Crit Care Med 2015;43(9):1964–77.

47. Milic MM, Puntillo K, Turner K, et al. Communicating with patients' families and physicians about prognosis and goals of care. Am J Crit Care 2015;24(4):e56–64.

48. Kahn JM, Le TQ, Barnato AE, et al. ICU telemedicine and critical care mortality: a National effectiveness study. Med Care 2016;54(3):319–25.

49. Lilly CM, Motzkus C, Rincon T, et al. ICU Telemedicine program financial outcomes. Chest 2017;151(2):286–97.

50. Kleinpell R, Barden C, Rincon T, et al. Assessing the impact of telemedicine on nursing care in intensive care units. Am J Crit Care 2016;25(1):e14–20.

51. Williams LS, Johnson E, Armaignac DL, et al. A mixed methods study of tele-ICU nursing interventions to prevent failure to rescue of patients in critical care. Telemed J E Health 2019;25(5):369–79.

52. Arneson SL, Tucker SJ, Mercier M, et al. Answering the call: impact of tele-ICU nurses during the COVID-19 pandemic. Crit Care Nurse 2020;40(4):25–31.

53. Morandi A, Brummel NE, Ely EW. Sedation, delirium and mechanical ventilation: the 'ABCDE' approach. Curr Opin Crit Care 2011;17(1):43–9.

54. Ely EW. The ABCDEF bundle: science and philosophy of how ICU liberation serves patients and families. Crit Care Med 2017;45(2):321–30.

55. Barnes-Daly MA, Pun BT, Harmon LA, et al. Improving health care for critically ill patients using an evidence-based collaborative approach to ABCDEF bundle dissemination and implementation. Worldviews Evid Based Nurs 2018;15(3):206–16.

56. Pun BT, Balas MC, Barnes-Daly MA, et al. Caring for critically ill patients with the ABCDEF bundle: results of the ICU liberation collaborative in over 15,000 adults. Crit Care Med 2019;47(1):3–14.

57. Hsieh SJ, Otusanya O, Gershengorn HB, et al. Staged implementation of awakening and breathing, coordination, delirium monitoring and management, and early mobilization bundle improves patient outcomes and reduces hospital costs. Crit Care Med 2019;47(7):885–93.

58. Barnes-Daly MA, Phillips G, Ely EW. Improving hospital survival and reducing brain dysfunction at seven California community hospitals: implementing PAD guidelines via the ABCDEF bundle in 6,064 patients. Crit Care Med 2017;45(2):171–8.

59. Balas MC, Devlin JW, Verceles AC, et al. Adapting the ABCDEF bundle to meet the needs of patients requiring prolonged mechanical ventilation in the long-term acute care hospital setting: historical perspectives and practical implications. Semin Respir Crit Care Med 2016;37(1):119–35.

60. Costa DK, Valley TS, Miller MA, et al. ICU team composition and its association with ABCDE implementation in a quality collaborative. J Crit Care 2018;44:1–6.

61. Boehm LM, Dietrich MS, Vasilevskis EE, et al. Perceptions of workload burden and adherence to ABCDE bundle among intensive care providers. Am J Crit Care 2017;26(4):e38–47.

62. Boltey EM, Iwashyna TJ, Hyzy RC, et al. Ability to predict team members' behaviors in ICU teams is associated with routine ABCDE implementation. J Crit Care 2019;51:192–7.

63. Boehm LM, Vasilevskis EE, Dietrich MS, et al. Organizational domains and variation in attitudes of intensive care providers toward the ABCDE bundle. Am J Crit Care 2017;26(3):e18–28.

64. Rhodes A, Evans LE, Alhazzani W, et al. Surviving sepsis campaign: international guidelines for management of sepsis and septic shock: 2016. Intensive Care Med 2017;43:304–77.

65. Kleinpell R, Blot S, Boulanger C, et al. International critical care nursing considerations and quality indicators for the 2017 surviving sepsis campaign guidelines. Intensive Care Med 2019;45(11):1663–6.

66. Furuya EY, Dick AW, Herzig CT, et al. Central line-associated bloodstream infection reduction and bundle compliance in intensive care units: a national study. Infect Control Hosp Epidemiol 2016;37(7):805–10.

67. Exline MC, Ali NA, Zikri N, et al. Beyond the bundle–journey of a tertiary care medical intensive care unit to zero central line-associated bloodstream infections. Crit Care 2013;17(2):R41.

68. Perin DC, Erdmann AL, Higashi GD, et al. Evidence-based measures to prevent central line-associated bloodstream infections: a systematic review. Rev Lat Am Enfermagem 2016;24:e2787.

69. Rosenthal VD, Bijie H, Maki DG, et al. International nosocomial infection control consortium (INICC) report, data summary of 36 countries, for 2004–2009. Am J Infect Control 2012;40(5):396–407.

70. Timsit JF, Esaied W, Neuville M, et al. Update on ventilator-associated pneumonia. F1000Res 2017;6:2061.

71. Ruppel H, De Vaux L, Cooper D, et al. Testing physiologic monitor alarm customization software to reduce alarm rates and improve nurses' experience of alarms in a medical intensive care unit. PLoS One 2018;13(10):e0205901.

72. Chlan LL, Savik K. Contributors to fatigue in patients receiving mechanical ventilatory support: a descriptive correlational study. Intensive Crit Care Nurs 2015; 31(5):303–8.

73. Glass D, Huang DT, Dugum M, et al. Rectal trumpet-associated hemorrhage in the intensive care unit: a quality improvement initiative. J Wound Ostomy Continence Nurs 2018;45(6):516–20.

74. Boev C, Xue Y, Ingersoll GL. Nursing job satisfaction, certification and healthcare-associated infections in critical care. Intensive Crit Care Nurs 2015;31(5):276–84.

75. Woodward BC, Umberger RA. Unit-level changes in central line-associated bloodstream infection before and after implementation of the affordable care act and mandatory reporting legislation. Dimens Crit Care Nurs 2018;37(1): 35–43.

76. Yakusheva O, Costa DK, Bobay KL, et al. Variability in catheter-associated asymptomatic bacteriuria rates among individual nurses in intensive care units: an observational cross-sectional study. PLoS One 2019;14(7):e0218755.

77. Morris PE, Berry MJ, Files DC, et al. Standardized rehabilitation and hospital length of stay among patients with acute respiratory failure: a randomized clinical trial. JAMA 2016;315(24):2694–702.

78. Stehman CR, Moromizato T, McKane CK, et al. Association between blood alcohol concentration and mortality in critical illness. J Crit Care 2015;30(6): 1382–9.

79. Jentzer JC, Anavekar NS, Brenes-Salazar JA, et al. Admission Braden skin score independently predicts mortality in cardiac intensive care patients. Mayo Clin Proc 2019;94(10):1994–2003.

80. D'Andrea MS, Fisichella PM. Improvement of postoperative pain control processes and outcomes in veterans of a surgical intensive care unit. World J Surg 2017;41(2):419–22.

81. Smit I, Harrison L, Letzkus L, et al. What factors are associated with the development of pressure ulcers in a medical intensive care unit? Dimens Crit Care Nurs 2016;35(1):37–41.
82. Hevener S, Rickabaugh B, Marsh T. Using a decision wheel to reduce use of restraints in a medical-surgical intensive care unit. Am J Crit Care 2016;25(6):479–86.
83. Knauert MP, Pisani M, Redeker N, et al. Pilot study: an intensive care unit sleep promotion protocol. BMJ Open Respir Res 2019;6(1):e000411.
84. Ding Q, Redeker NS, Pisani MA, et al. Factors influencing patients' sleep in the intensive care unit: perceptions of patients and clinical staff. Am J Crit Care 2017;26(4):278–86.
85. American Association of Colleges of Nursing. AACN position statement on nursing research. Washington, DC: American Association of Colleges of Nursing; 2006. p. 1–16. Available at: https://www.aacnnursing.org/News-Information/Position-Statements-White-Papers/Nursing-Research. Accessed October 3, 2020.
86. Girard TD, Exline MC, Carson SS, et al. Haloperidol and ziprasidone for treatment of delirium in critical illness. N Engl J Med 2018;379(26):2506–16.
87. Kotfis K, Marra A, Ely EW. ICU delirium - a diagnostic and therapeutic challenge in the intensive care unit. Anaesthesiol Intensive Ther 2018;50(2):160–7.
88. Dubb R, Nydahl P, Hermes C, et al. Barriers and strategies for early mobilization of patients in intensive care units. Ann Am Thorac Soc 2016;13(5):724–30.
89. Jo M, Song MK, Knafl GJ, et al. Family-clinician communication in the ICU and its relationship to psychological distress of family members: a cross-sectional study. Int J Nurs Stud 2019;95:34–9.
90. Udelsman BV, Lee KC, Traeger LN, et al. Clinician-to-clinician communication of patient goals of care within a surgical intensive care unit. J Surg Res 2019;240:80–8.
91. Fusaro MV, Becker C, Scurlock C. Evaluating Tele-ICU implementation based on observed and predicted ICU mortality: a systematic review and meta-analysis. Crit Care Med 2019;47(4):501–7.

Caring for Traumatic Brain Injury Patients
Australian Nursing Perspectives

Vicki Evans, RN, GDip Neuroscience, Management[a,b,*]

KEYWORDS

• TBI • Concussion • Head injury • Neuroscience nursing

KEY POINTS

- Management of traumatic brain injury (TBI) requires prompt neurologic assessment among a highly specialized multidisciplinary team of health practitioners for the best possible patient outcome.
- Most people experiencing mild TBI recover fully within days to months, but a small percentage of individuals continue to experience symptoms 3 months or more after injury.
- Recognition and management of concussion have become major health concerns across all sport arenas, from professional sport to school sport and backyard games.

INTRODUCTION—AUSTRALIAN HEALTH CARE

Australia is the world's sixth largest country after Russia, Canada, China, the United States and Brazil, equating to approximately 5% of the world's land area, and is the world's largest island.[1] Australia is made up of 6 states and 1 territory and has a current population of 25,415,000.[2] Large transport distances are inherent to the Australian geography. The Royal Flying Doctor Service[3] founded in 1928, is one of the largest and most comprehensive aeromedical organizations in the world, providing extensive primary health care and 24-hour emergency service to people over an area of 7.69 million km².

Health care expenditure across most health systems is growing at a great rate, which is attributable to the increasing demand for health care services due to aging populations and the increased burden of chronic disease, continued advances in medical technology, and ever-growing community expectations. Australia has universal health cover and the health system consists of a mix of public and private sector

[a] World Federation of Neuroscience Nurses; [b] Neuroscience, Royal North Shore Hospital, Pacific Highway, St. Leonard's, Sydney, New South Wales 2065, Australia
* Level 7 (7D) Royal North Shore Hospital, Pacific Highway, St Leonards, NSW 2065, Australia.
E-mail address: Vicki.Evans@health.nsw.gov.au

Crit Care Nurs Clin N Am 33 (2021) 21–36
https://doi.org/10.1016/j.cnc.2020.10.002   ccnursing.theclinics.com
0899-5885/21/Crown Copyright © 2020 Published by Elsevier Inc. All rights reserved.

health services, financed through a combination of income tax, a specific income levy (the Medicare Levy) and private financing by individuals through private health insurance premiums and out-of-pocket payments.

There is a high resource requirement associated with patients with TBI. Patients with brain injuries generally have extended intensive care unit and hospital stays. Evidence-based guidelines concerning systemic monitoring and supportive measures are utilized in TBI care.[4]

Like all other countries, Australia is seeing an increase in traumatic brain injuries (TBIs) from a variety of causes—road trauma, sporting events, blast injuries, combat injuries, and falls and trauma at school or in the backyard. **Box 1** describes head injury definitions. When discussing TBI, the mechanics behind force need to be understood and can be explained with Newton's laws of motion.[5] Gravitational is the force of gravity on a particular body—a measurement of acceleration (g) that causes the perception of weight.[6] The force of gravity while standing on the earth is $1g$, and this increases markedly if slapped on the back to approximately $4.1g$, then further when in a car or a rollercoaster, and even more if having sustained a concussion ($80g$–$100g$).[6,7]

TBI is an acute brain injury resulting from a blow to the head from external forces.[8] It is a major cause of lifelong disability and death worldwide but is considered a silent epidemic because society is largely unaware of the magnitude of the problem. Sporting injuries are a large group where TBI, in particular concussion, is apparent. Intense media coverage of affected footballers has saturated television screens and movie theaters since the National Football League became embroiled in legal cases concerning players with chronic traumatic encephalopathy (CTE).[9] As a consequence, other sporting codes across the globe have met and adopted strategies to identify and monitor players for concussion and implement guidelines for player welfare, not only in elite sports but also school sports as well.

TBI patterns have changed over the past decades, with an aging population resulting in higher numbers of fall-related injuries.[10] The Australian Institute of Health and Welfare reported a TBI rate of 295/100,000 population.[11] Most studies suggest that approximately 20% of patients with TBI admitted to the hospital have sustained moderate or severe head injuries, and the other 80% have mild injuries. Early multidisciplinary involvement is required. Access to services and support, however, can be limited depending on socioeconomic, geographic, environmental, and cultural factors.[12] One study showed that TBI due to assault was 21 times more likely in Aboriginal and Torres Strait Islander peoples compared with non-Indigenous Australians.[13] TBI is a complex injury with a broad spectrum of symptoms and disabilities, including physical, mental, cognitive, and social problems.

TBIs can include scalp lacerations, skull fractures, extradural hematoma (EDH), subdural hematoma (SDH), diffuse axonal injury, intracerebral hemorrhage (ICH), traumatic subarachnoid hemorrhage, intraventricular hemorrhage (IVH), and concussion.

MECHANISM OF INJURY

TBI occurs from acceleration or deceleration forces—including a blow to the head that can cause laceration of the scalp, skull fracture, and/or shifting of the intracranial contents, with resultant focal and/or diffuse changes.[14,15] Focal changes include hematoma formation resulting from tearing of blood vessels, and contusion or bruising, most commonly on the basal and polar portions of the frontal and temporal lobes. Complications, including brain swelling, infection, raised intracranial pressure (ICP), and respiratory arrest, may cause secondary brain injury. TBI can be classified in several ways, as shown in **Box 2**.

Box 1
Definitions used in head injury

Condition	Definition
Contusion	Focal bruising of brain tissue; frequently occurs near the site of a skull fracture
Concussion	A complex pathophysiologic process affecting the brain, induced by traumatic biomechanical forces
	Reversible physiologic change in nervous system function without a gross anatomic abnormality Consciousness is lost or impaired and retrograde or anterograde amnesia (or both) may occur. No focal deficit usually is present.
Laceration	Usually involves tearing of brain tissue and often associated with depressed skull fractures or open head injuries
Skull fracture	A break or split in the skull, as a result of trauma to the head
Depressed skull fracture	A fracture with inward displacement of a part of the calvarium (skull) onto the brain
EDH	Bleeding (usually arterial) between the skull and dura, almost always associated with a linear skull fracture. Because the dura becomes adherent to the skull with age, EDH rarely is seen in the elderly. Treatment is a craniotomy to relieve pressure to prevent herniation and to stop the bleeding.
SDH	Bleeding (usually venous) between the dura and arachnoid layers. SDH can be located anywhere within the cranial cavity, but it is seen most frequently over the convexity. Presentation can be days to weeks postinjury. Treatment usually is via a burr hole.
Intracerebral hemorrhage	Hemorrhage >5 mL within the brain matter
Traumatic subarachnoid hemorrhage	Traumatic subarachnoid hemorrhage usually requires no surgery because the blood is within the subarachnoid space spreads into the CSF. There is an association, however, of poorer outcome with traumatic subarachnoid hemorrhage.
Intraventricular hemorrhage	Bleeding within the ventricles may occur following trauma or subarachnoid hemorrhage.
ICP	The Monro-Kellie hypothesis states that the skull is a rigid box. Inside, there are 3 noncompressible components (brain, blood, and CSF). If one increases in size, then the others need to decrease to compensate. If this does not happen, then a buildup of pressure within the skull develops, leading to herniation syndromes.
Burr hole	A small opening in the skull made with a surgical drill
Craniotomy	Surgery involving removal of the skull bone to gain access to the brain and the bone is put back in place.
Craniectomy	A surgery to remove skull bone to allow for brain swelling and reduce intracranial hypertension. The removed pieces of bone are reinserted months later, when the swelling is resolved.
PTA	Loss of memory for events immediately following a trauma. The patient is confused and disoriented and day-to-day memory is unreliable.
CSF leak	Rhinorrhea—CSF leaking out the nose; otorrhea—CSF leaking out the ear

> **Box 2**
> **Traumatic brain injury classification**[14–16]
>
> - Mild head injury—classified as a GCS of 13 to 15 on admission
> - Moderate head injury—classified as a GCS of 9 to 12 on admission
> - Severe head injury—classified as a GCS of 3 to 8 on admission
>
> TBI can also be grouped into
>
> - Open head injury
> - Closed head injury

TBI predominates in young men, most commonly associated with high-speed motor vehicle accidents, and in elderly patients suffering falls. Public health measures to prevent and reduce the severity of initial injuries together with strategies to minimize secondary brain injuries are likely to be of key importance in improving outcomes from TBI.[17] Australia was the first country to make wearing bicycle helmets mandatory in the early 1990s, making a difference in the severity of head injury.[18]

Most people experiencing mild TBI recover fully within days to months, but a small percentage of individuals continue to experience symptoms 3 months after injury. Recovery from moderate or severe TBI tends to follow a negatively accelerating curve, which is most rapid in the first 3 months to 6 months, but may continue for several years.[19]

MANAGEMENT OF TRAUMATIC BRAIN INJURY IN AUSTRALIAN EMERGENCY DEPARTMENTS

Australian evidence-based guidelines for the management of TBI in the emergency department (ED) are widely available.[20–23] Computerized tomography (CT) is the criterion standard for diagnosing TBI, with magnetic resonance imaging (MRI) used to detect structural changes in moderate-to-severe TBI.[24] Yet, although CT identifies TBIs rapidly and accurately, potentially reducing morbidity and mortality, it is costly, requires patients to cooperate and lie still, and exposes patients to radiation.[25,26] It, therefore, is paramount that clinicians, medical and nursing, have appropriate assessment skills and the ability to navigate and make sense of these available tools (**Box 3**).

GLASGOW COMA SCALE

The Glasgow Coma Scale (GCS) is a standardized tool that is used worldwide to assess neurologic status.[27] Clinical judgment and reviewing the GCS and the posttraumatic amnesia (PTA) assessments give clinicians an idea of how well a patient is neurologically.

POSTTRAUMATIC AMNESIA

Posttraumatic amnesia (PTA) is the period of time following head injury in which a patient is disorientated or confused. There is a short-term memory dysfunction. It can last for hours, days, or longer depending on the severity of injury. The duration of PTA is an important index of the severity of head injury and the length of time in PTA is more significant than the length of time unconscious.[27,28] PTA assessment is to commence in ED for patients with a TBI. It is a screening device and must be used in conjunction with clinical judgment.[29] The Westmead Post-Traumatic Amnesia

---

Box 3
Emergency department considerations for traumatic brain injury patients[20–22]

- Always suspect a cervical spine injury until proved otherwise.
- Loss of consciousness (witnessed) at the scene?
- Wearing a helmet?
- Wearing a mouth guard?
- Is there a CSF leak?
- Cranial nerves
- Motor/sensory
- Speech
- Exclude hypoglycemia as cause for neurologic deterioration.
- Look for other injuries
- CT scan

Scale (WPTAS) and the Abbreviated WPTAS (A-WPTAS) are validated tools for use with TBI patients,[27–32] looking at cognitive safety following head injury. The A-WPTAS also includes the GCS and is an objective measure of PTA for use in the ED.[28,31] It is to be done hourly for 4 hours or until the goal score of 18/18 is reached, indicating that the individual is out of PTA. If the patient is admitted, the daily PTA scale must be utilized instead of the A-WPTAS and the patient must score 12/12 on 3 consecutive days. Therefore, this may mean that the patient is admitted for a minimum of 3 days. The PTA assessment allows for an accurate review of memory ability after head injury and completes the package of the patient for the local general practitioner to follow.[27] All staff are required to successfully master a computer education program prior to assessing patients for PTA.

Mortimer and Berg[33] describe agitation in patients recovering from TBI and the appropriate nursing management, including multifaceted assessments, individualized patient care plans, quiet environment, and limited stimuli (visitors, procedures, room allocation, and noise). These patients require a level of care that includes constant observation and safety checks. It is important that they, where possible, are housed close to the nurses' station for observation and that they are given short responses because attention span and ability to retain information usually are impaired.

CONCUSSION

Concussion is a head injury that may cause instant loss of awareness or alertness for a few minutes to a few hours after a TBI.[27,30,34] Concussion now is thought to be of greater significance particularly for school-aged children, and they should not be playing sport until they are completely symptom-free.[34–37] Head injuries are an inherent risk of participating in contact sport. Concussion occurs, however, in the home and schoolyard as well.

Concussion reflects a functional injury to the brain. Clinical features generally are short-lived and resolve spontaneously, usually within 10 days to 14 days. Adolescents, however, may take longer to recover (3–4 weeks) and require longer time off school and sport.[38] It is important to make a clinical diagnosis of concussion from structural head injury, estimate the severity of the injury, and determine when a graded return to school or work can commence. After clinical features have resolved and no analgesia is being consumed, then a graded return to sport can be considered.[34]

A careful history, including time of injury, mechanism of injury, loss of consciousness, seizure activity, GCS, and observation, is required for all head knocks. Postconcussive symptoms frequently occur and parents should be aware of what to expect and the duration. Regular follow-up until all symptoms have resolved is required.[35]

Early diagnosis and appropriate management of individuals who have sustained a TBI facilitate good outcomes. Evidence now suggests that the cumulative effects of repeated concussions increase the likelihood of cognitive impairment later in life. Once a person has had a concussion, he/she is as much as 4 times more likely to sustain a second one. Moreover, after several concussions, it takes less of a blow to cause the injury and requires more time to recover.[37]

SECOND IMPACT SYNDROME

Young brains are particularly susceptible to second impact syndrome, which results from acute, usually fatal, cerebral edema thought to be from the loss of cerebral autoregulation.[37] This occurs when a second concussion is sustained before there is complete recovery from the first concussion. It is thought to be almost completely preventable. Therefore, education must center on reporting the injury.

ADOLESCENTS AND CONCUSSION

A more conservative approach to concussion management should be taken with those ages 18 years or younger.[39–44] Developmental milestone networks easily are damaged in adolescents after a head knock and typically they have a longer recovery trajectory of 3-4 weeks, compared to 7-10 days for children or adults.[38,40] There is a commonality with migraine, making symptoms worse. In adolescents, headache, vestibular symptoms, and neck pain are common, with reports of fatigue and exercise intolerance in postconcussive syndromes.

Whereas rest once was thought to be the mainstay for concussion treatment, rest now is thought to be important in the acute phase (first 24–48 hours) only, with increasing exercise after that time.[36–38] Adding activities slowly and evaluating symptoms are key to recovery. Education regarding the importance of reporting symptoms is required for the individual, family, teachers, coaches, and managers. Neck strengthening exercises are an important routine. The quality of the neck muscles can help stabilize the rebound effects of a head knock.[43]

The international Concussion in Sport group (CISG)[37] have met several times over the past decade to formulate and discuss guidelines for the management of concussion in sport. From the Berlin meeting in 2016,[37] it was stated that the strongest and most consistent predictor of slower recovery from sports-related concussion is the severity of a person's initial symptoms in the first day, or initial few days, after injury. There is some evidence that the teenage years, in particular, the high school years, are the most vulnerable for having persistent symptoms—with greater risk for girls than boys. Under-reporting of concussion still is a problem. Education to improve knowledge and understanding of the condition is required. Legislation alone is ineffective. Athletes themselves need to have a good understanding of concussion in order to appreciate the importance of reporting symptoms and complying with rest and return to sport advice. Parents and coaches also must be able to recognize the symptoms and signs of concussion. Slogans, such as "If in doubt-Sit it out" and "It's better to miss 1 game than the whole season," are a good start to give an understanding of the ramifications of poorly treated concussions (CISG).[37] Concussed children must not return to sport until they have successfully resumed normal school activities, without aggravating their symptoms.[37,44]

Most sporting organizations and schools now have mandated guidelines that cover concussion definition, removal from play, sideline testing, and a stepwise return-to-play protocol. There are, however, loopholes in which players can hide symptoms in order to play. Hiding symptoms is suboptimal and requires repetitive education steps.[44,45]

CT scan—look for **SYMMETRY**. Then look at

- **BLOOD**: inspect the brain for any signs of bleeding.
- **CISTERNS**: examine the cisterns. Are they all open; any compression?
- **BRAIN**: evaluate the brain parenchyma. Are there any masses, contusions, or midline shift?
- **VENTRICLES**: evaluate the ventricles. Are they symmetric and size normal?
- **BONE**: evaluate the bone. Are there any skull fractures or hyperostosis; is the skull shape normal? Bone has the highest density on CT scan (whitest in appearance.) Evaluate for fracture.

CONSIDERATIONS FOR MANAGING A PATIENT WITH A TRAUMATIC BRAIN INJURY
Neurologic Assessment—Glasgow Coma Scale, Posttraumatic Amnesia, Vital Signs

Frequent and accurate neurologic assessment is warranted in the TBI setting.[20–23,34] Observing a patient, not necessarily with machines but rather with the eyes for any differing signs is important in order to identify any small changes quickly and take appropriate measures for the best outcome. Early detection of a change in status of a neurologic patient improves the prognosis. In the TBI patient, it also is prudent to be aware of other conditions that may interfere with an accurate assessment, including drugs, alcohol, age, and other injuries. Changes in the neurologic status of the TBI patient can be extremely quick or relatively slow. The first and main change is in level of consciousness.

Early neurologic findings
- Decreased level of consciousness
- Crow's feet, wrinkles on 1 side of the face but not the other
- Headache
- Extremity drift
- Sluggish pupils
Later neurologic signs
- Continued deterioration in level of consciousness
- Worsening headache
- Hemiplegia
- Vomiting
- Decorticate/decerebrate posturing
- Decreased cough, gag, and/or corneal reflexes
- Change in vital signs or Cushing triad (widening pulse pressure, bradycardia, and irregular respirations)
- Pupils—unequal or no response to light

Neurological observations - including GCS, cranial nerve testing, PTA score and vital signs are the mainstay of a thorough neurological assessment. These are dependent on the severity of injury and whether the patient is managed in the ED, intensive care unit, or neurosurgical ward. If the GCS differs by 1 point, this requires a clinical review but may be related to assessment technique. If the GCS differs by 2 points, however, a rapid response is required from the neurosurgical team. Some patients require hourly observations, but these should be done in an acute-care or high-dependency setting. They may be warranted for a short duration, for example, hourly for 4 hours in a ward setting. Nevertheless, and irrespective of where a patient is housed, minimum observations should include neurologic and vital signs at least every 4 hours, unless otherwise charted (**Box 4**).

Airway Management

- Hypoxemia—avoid and/or correct.
- Optimize oxygenation and ensure patent airway.
- Use supplemental oxygen to keep arterial oxygen saturation greater than 95% and Pao_2 greater than 80 mm Hg.[46]
- Consider intubation and mechanical ventilation (GCS <8, requires endotracheal intubation).
- Many patients may be combative and require sedation for cervical spine control. In this setting, endotracheal intubation may be the best course of management.

Blood Pressure Management

- Fluid resuscitation with 0.9% sodium chloride should be administered as appropriate to the volume status of the patient to avoid/limit hypotension.
- Vasopressors, antihypertensives, and vasodilator agents may be considered.
- All sedatives and anesthetic agents can precipitate hypotension. If hypotension occurs, sedative agents must be reduced or suspended until blood pressure is maintained.

Control Intracranial Pressure and Prevention of Increased Intracranial Pressure

- Keep ICP less than 20 mm Hg and cerebral perfusion pressure greater than 60.
- Positioning: routinely, head of bed at 30° (if other injuries allow)
- Environment—limit visitors to 2 per visit; quiet room.
- Medications—pain management, osmotic diuretics, barbiturates
- Brain Trauma Foundation (2016)[4]—steroids are not recommended for improving outcome or reducing ICP.

Box 4 Neurologic assessments	
Regardless of the Diagnosis, Neurologic Assessment Is the same	Neuroscience Nurses Should Possess the Necessary Skills that Allow Them To
Vital signs	Observe
GCS	Examine
Cranial nerves	Question
Motor/sensory	Assess
Proprioception	Treat
Document	Document

- Although propofol is recommended for the control of ICP, it does not decrease mortality or improve outcome at 6 months.[47]

Medications

- Pain management: provision of analgesia for head injury is complex because
  1. The assessment of a patient's mental state is used as a routine measure of either improvement or decline in neurologic function. Medications that alter the sensorium or cause sedation, such as opioid analgesics, can interfere with such assessment.
  2. Drugs that decrease the respiratory response to arterial carbon dioxide (such as opioids) can result in reduced alveolar ventilation and hypercarbia, which can increase cerebral blood flow, worsen cerebral edema, and raise ICP.
  3. Some medications have a constipating effect, which can increase ICP. Aperients should be administered.

Drugs to be avoided
Tramadol hydrochloride and nonsteroidal anti-inflammatory drugs are effective analgesics and essentially nonsedating. Side effects (seizure and interference with platelet function), however, make them unsuitable in the head-injured patient. Paracetamol (acetaminophen) is the exception because it does not interfere with platelet function.
The most important things to remember about analgesia are the following:

- Analgesia aims at pain control, not total abolition of pain.
- Take an accurate medical history, including allergies and pain history.
- Ensure accurate assessment of pain.
- Monitor sedation score.
- Review effect of analgesia.
- Use caution with hepatotoxic risk factors.
- Consider patient's renal function status.
- Use caution with pediatrics, adolescents, and the elderly.

Other medications to consider

- Pneumovax—if cerebrospinal fluid (CSF) leak or basilar skull fracture, to prevent meningitis
- Tetanus—check status
- Mannitol or hypertonic saline, if ICP is elevated
- Phenobarbitone

Antiseizure prophylaxis
The incidence of seizures after penetrating head injuries is between 30% and 50%. In closed head injuries, the risk is somewhat lower. There is no level I evidence, however, to support that treatment with prophylactic anticonvulsants reduces the occurrence of late seizures or has any effect on death or neurologic morbidity.[4]
Certain risk factors place patients in a higher category for developing posttraumatic seizures, including GCS less than 10, cortical contusion, depressed skull fracture, SDH, EDH, intracranial hemorrhage, penetrating head wound, and seizure within 24 hours of injury. Antiepileptics may be used to prevent the occurrence of seizures in high-risk patients during the first week after TBI. Routine seizure prophylaxis beyond 1 week, however, is not recommended.

Surgery

- Evacuation of the hematoma via burr hole or craniotomy.

- Some hemorrhages may be monitored and have deliberate delayed surgery or be managed medically without surgery, depending on their presentation.
- Decompressive surgery: may have benefits in severe TBI with raised ICP.
- Depressed skull fractures: compound skull fractures usually have surgery to prevent infection and require antibiotics.
- Closed depressed skull fractures may be managed nonoperatively.
- Hypothermia: there currently is no evidence to support that routine hypothermia is beneficial in the treatment of TBI.

The Multidisciplinary Team

The multidisciplinary team is a treatment team approach to meet the complex needs of the neurosurgical patient recovering from TBI. It begins from the moment a patient is allocated to the neurosurgical service and consists of a neurosurgeon, neurosurgical nurses, physiotherapist, occupational therapist, speech therapist, social worker, dietitian, neuropsychologist, and rehabilitation specialist. In most regions of Australia, there are specialized brain injury rehabilitation services that accept referrals for people with persisting disability after TBI. The effects of severe TBI are long-lasting, and patients and their families require continued care and support, often for the rest of their lives.

TBI is most prevalent in young adult life and often disrupts important developmental processes, such as attaining independence from parental support, completing study, establishing a vocation/returning to work, and forming social networks. Therefore, this can result in a loss of self-esteem, social withdrawal, and a considerable hardship for families, with challenging behavior, potential for hazardous drug and alcohol use, mental health problems, and housing and employment issues. The National Disability Insurance Scheme[48] is intended to provide lifetime care and support to all Australians and their families/carers with a permanent and significant disability, aged under 65, who sustain a catastrophic injury from a motor vehicle, workplace, medical treatment injury. or general accident.

Case Study

A case study is shown in **Box 5**.

DISCHARGE FOLLOWING TRAUMATIC BRAIN INJURY FROM THE EMERGENCY DEPARTMENT OR WARD

Cognitive impairments represent the greatest challenge following TBI and the impact on the patient and family dynamics postinjury is great.

- Patients with a history of loss of consciousness or amnesia post–head injury must be observed for a minimum of 4 hours in an ED or ward prior to discharge.
- Patients with any intermediate risk or continuing symptoms must be admitted for further observation.
- The multidisciplinary team (including medical, nursing, and allied health members) ensures a collaborative approach to discharge. Referrals should be made early for streamlined care. The MDT should also include consultation with the patient's family to ensure ongoing supervision.
- PTA testing is complete and satisfactory for discharge.

Prior to discharge, the following criteria must be met and assessed by a medical registrar or specialist:

- Consciousness has recovered fully.

Box 5
Case study

10:00 PM, July 2016 (July in Australia is midwinter and dark at 6:00 PM)
- A 15-year-old boy presents to an ED with a 4-hour history of "bad" headache.
- Academic family
- Currently in year 10; examination week
- Given paracetamol ×4 at 6:00 PM as well as aspirin, 300 mg, at home
- No neurologic deficits other than headache
- Vital signs—normal
- No other information recorded in patient notes
- Had CT, MRI, angiogram—all normal
- Length of stay = 4 days

Questions that should have been asked on admission:

What were you doing when your headache came on?
   A: Computer work for my examinations.

You are wearing glasses. Do you normally wear them?
   A: Yes

Were you wearing them when your headache started?
   A: No. I do not like wearing them.

It is dark at that time of night. Did you have a light on?
   A: No. I was just using the backlight from the computer.

Do you normally take paracetamol and aspirin for headache?
   A: No. I took paracetamol but it did not work, so I took aspirin half hour later. I needed to study.

Concerns: Lack of questioning initiated a CT, MRI, invasive angiogram, and a 4-day length of stay...to diagnose eye strain. This had an impact on the patient, family, their costs, and hospital bed and resource implications.

- The patient is eating and drinking normally with no vomiting.
- Neurologic symptoms either have resolved or are minor and resolving.
- The patient either is self-caring or returning to a safe environment with suitable social support.
- The results of imaging and other investigations have been reviewed and no further investigations are required.
- There are no other injuries.

Social criteria to be met prior to discharge at home with observation:

- Responsible parent/guardian is available and willing to observe the patient for at least 24 hours.
- Verbal and written instructions and discharge advice about observations and actions are discussed with the parent/guardian.
- Home is within reasonable access to medical advice and easy access to telephone
- Transportation home is available.
- Standard written discharge information is to be provided

Follow-up is to include

- Letter to the patient's general practitioner
- Verbal and written discharge instructions

And may require

- Specific TBI appointment for further management
- Pediatric outpatient clinic appointment
- Letter to the child's school—standardized concussion school letter
- Neurosurgical outpatient clinic appointment
- Neuropsychological referral

Concussion Summary

- Check mechanism of injury.
- Check short-term memory.
- "If in doubt, sit it out."
- "It's better to miss 1 game than the whole season."

How can parents be encouraged to let their children play a contact sport (rugby) knowing that memory issues after repeated concussions CTE might be their fate?

- CTE should not be used as a scare tactic.
- Rule changes and enforcement of rules have improved recognition and management of on-field concussion.
- Encourage fair play and sportsman-like behavior.
- Encourage mouth guards and headgear.
- Encourage reporting of symptoms and importance of not playing with symptoms.
- Encourage Sport Concussion Assessment Tool[36,37] tests preseason, during season, and postseason.
- Encourage importance of looking for a head knock and mechanism of injury.
- Encourage removing the player from play if head knock occurred.
- Lead by example.

Why do animals, such as woodpeckers or bighorn sheep, not get concussions?

Zhu and colleagues[49] described bighorn sheep, as a part of fighting and mating, routinely experiencing violent impacts to the head without negative consequences to their brains or horns. Their horns consist of a bony material and a trabecular mesh-like structure, which absorbs the impact of ramming. The woodpecker also has significant internal structures, such as a secured hyoid bone, uneven beak, and tight cranial cavity, that absorb the impact of pecking a tree at more than 20 times per second.[49] In humans, mouth guards and helmets help absorb the impact of contact sport.

SUMMARY

To be overprotective, like being wrapped in cotton wool, is not an option. Sport and fun are synonymous and healthy, the world over. The desire to go fast is thrilling and it seems that the faster, the better! Keeping a child safe is a parent's obligation, and theme park operators, governments, and companies have that same obligation for public safety. Despite many safety procedures, however, device and equipment injury still occurs.

Although life is becoming a minefield of safe operating practices and every product has a warning attached, fun activities are encouraged, just within reason. The brain, within its hardened case, is protected but also vulnerable to changes in pressure and force. Preexisting brain or neck conditions, whether known or not, play a role in injury from innocuous day-to-day activities, schoolyard injury, sporting injury, motor vehicle accidents, and theme park rides. When participating in these activities and the pressure they place on the body, some obligation must rest with the individual. Their health and informed decision on whether or not to participate.

Education of the greater community, including schools and sporting clubs, is required. Making people aware of the choices in order to prevent, protect, and/or manage head injuries is essential. Neuroscience nurses are at the forefront of leading this education—through seminars and school educational sessions—covering prevention strategies, first-aid management on field, hospital management, and rehabilitation.

Early recognition and expert neurologic assessment are required for optimal patient management and recovery.

CLINICS CARE POINTS

- In order to impress upon the importance of timely identification and management of the concussed individual, the saying "It's better to miss one game, than the whole season" resonates well with children and young adults.
- Note: the intention regarding analgesia in a head-injured/neurosurgical patient is to make the patient comfortable and aims at pain control, not necessarily pain abolition.
- It is important to consider cranial anatomic defects, such as skull fractures, in particular those affecting the base of skull and extending to the sinuses and petrous pyramids.
- ALERT! Basal skull fracture: always think there may be a fracture of the base of skull if there is a CSF leak. This also should alert to the fact that if things are leaking out, then bugs can get in, leading to meningitis.
- AVOID nasogastric tubes or nasopharyngeal airways if a fractured base of skull is considered.
- Battle sign (bruising of the mastoid bone behind the ear) and/or raccoon eyes (bilateral periorbital bruising) are present with a fractured base of skull.

How to tell if it is a CSF leak?

- Look for the halo sign: drip CSF onto the white sheet or white gauze—a bluish ring appears if CSF is present. Collect a sample and send it to a laboratory for confirmation. (Note: dipstick for glucose is unreliable because glucose is present in blood.)
- Management: If there is a CSF leak—lay the patient 30° head up and place sterile white gauze over the ear (otorrhea) or under the nose (rhinorrhea). Monitor the amount.

DISCLOSURE

The author has nothing to disclose.

REFERENCES

1. Global Burden of Disease 2016 Traumatic Brain Injury and Spinal Cord Collaborators. Global, regional, and national burden of traumatic brain injury and spinal cord injury, 1990–2016: a systematic analysis for the Global Burden of Disease Study 2016. Lancet 2019;18:56–87.

2. Australian Bureau of Statistics. 2019. Available at: https://www.abs.gov.au/ausstats. Accessed November 26, 2019.

3. Royal Flying Doctor Service (RFDS). Available at: www.flyingdoctor.org.au. Accessed February 11, 2020.
4. Brain Trauma Foundation: American Association of Neurological Surgeons, Congress of Neurological Surgeons. Guidelines for the management of severe traumatic brain injury. 4th edition. 2016. Available at: www.braintrauma.org.
5. Newton's laws of motion. Available at: https://www.britannica.com/science/Newtons-laws-of-motion. Accessed February 13, 2020.
6. Slade S. Feel the G's – the science of gravity and G-forces. Mankato, MN: Compass Point Books; 2009. Accessed January 7, 2020. Available at: https://www.amazon.com/Feel-Gs-Science-G-Forces-Headline/dp/0756540526.
7. Beaudette D. Report on G-force effects on the human body. Virginia:: Department of Transportation, Federal Aviation Administration. National Technical Information Service, U.S. Department of Commerce; 1984.
8. WHO. Neurotrauma. 2004. Available at: https://www.who.int. Accessed November 27, 2019.
9. National Football League concussion Settlement. Available at: www.nflconcussionsettlement.com. Accessed October 20, 2019.
10. Roozenbeek B, Maas AI, Menon DK. Changing patterns in the epidemiology of traumatic brain injury. Nat Rev Neurol 2019;43(4):382–8.
11. Pozzato I, Tate L, Rosenkoetter U, et al. Epidemiology of hospitalised traumatic brain injury in the state of New South Wales, Australia: a population-based study. Aust N Z J Public Health 2019. https://doi.org/10.1111/1753-6405.12878.
12. Bohanna I, Fitts MS, Bird K, et al. The transition from hospital to home: protocol for a longitudinal study of Australian aboriginal and Torres Strait Islander traumatic brain injury (TBI). Brain Impairment 2018;19(3):246–57.
13. Jamieson LM, Harrison JE, Berry JG. Hospitalisation for head injury due to assault among Indigenous and non-Indigenous Australians, July 1999–June 2005. Med J Aust 2008;188:576–9.
14. Brain Trauma Foundation. Guidelines for the surgical management of traumatic brain injury. 4th edition. New York: Brain Trauma Foundation; 2016.
15. Carney N, Totten AM, O'Reilly C, et al. Guidelines for the management of severe traumatic brain injury, 4th edition. Neurosurgery 2017;80(1):6–15.
16. Available at: https://www.brainline.org/article/what-glasgow-coma-scale. Accessed November 27, 2019.
17. Myburgh JA, Cooper D, James MD, et al. Epidemiology and 12-month outcomes from traumatic brain injury in Australia and New Zealand. J Trauma 2008;64(4):854–62.
18. Oliver J, Creighton P. Bicycle injuries and helmet use: a systematic review and meta-analysis. Int J Epidemiol 2017;46(1):372.
19. Cramer SC, Sur M, Dobkin BH, et al. Harnessing neuroplasticity for clinical applications. Brain 2011;134:1591–609.
20. Reed D. Adult trauma clinical practice guidelines, initial management of closed head injury in adults, 2nd edition summary report. North Sydney: NSW Institute of Trauma and Injury Management. NSW Health; 2011.
21. NSW Ministry of health initial management of closed head injury in adults 2nd edition PD2013. Available at: https://www.aci.health.nsw.gov.au/__data/assets/pdf_file/0003/195150/Closed_Head_Injury_CPG_2nd_Ed_Full_document.pdf. Accessed October 7, 2019.
22. NSW Health - Acute management of head injury in children within the first 24 hours. Available at: https://www1.health.nsw.gov.au/pds/ActivePDSDocuments/PD2012_013.pdf. Accessed October 7, 2019.

23. Available at: https://braintrauma.org/uploads/03/12/Guidelines_for_Management_of_Severe_TBI_4th_Edition.pdf. Accessed November 26, 2019.

24. Arciniegas DB, Anderson CA, Topkoff J, et al. Mild traumatic brain injury: a neuropsychiatric approach to diagnosis, evaluation, and treatment. Neuropsychiatr Dis Treat 2005;1:311–27.

25. Brenner DJ, Hall EJ. Computed tomography–an increasing source of radiation exposure. N Engl J Med 2007;357(22):2277–84.

26. Pearce MS, Salotti JA, Little MP, et al. Radiation exposure from CT scans in childhood and subsequent risk of leukaemia and brain tumours: a retrospective cohort study. Lancet 2012;380(9840):499–505.

27. Ponsford J, Cameron P, Wilmott C, et al. Use of the Westmead PTA scale to monitor recovery after mild head injury. Brain Inj 2004;18:603–14.

28. Shores EA, Lammél A, Hullick C, et al. The diagnostic accuracy of the Revised Westmead PTA Scale as an adjunct to the Glasgow Coma Scale in the early identification of cognitive impairment in patients with mild traumatic brain injury. J Neurol Neurosurg Psychiatry 2008;79:1100–6.

29. Bosch M, McKenzie JE, Ponsford JL, et al. Evaluation of a targeted, theory-informed implementation intervention designed to increase uptake of emergency management recommendations regarding adult patients with mild traumatic brain injury: results of the NET cluster randomised trial. Implement Sci 2019;14:4.

30. Ponsford J, Nguyen S, Downing M, et al. Factors associated with persistent post-concussion symptoms following mild traumatic brain injury in adults. J Rehabil Med 2019;51(1):32–9.

31. Watson CE, Clous EA, Jaeger M, D'amours SK. Introduction of the abbreviated Westmead post-traumatic amnesia scale and impact on length of stay. Scand J Surg 2017;106(4):356–60.

32. Shores EA. Further concurrent validity on the Westmead PTA scale. Appl Neuropsychol 1995;2:167–9.

33. Mortimer DS, Berg W. Agitation in patients recovering from traumatic brain injury nursing management. J Neurosci Nurs 2017;49(1):25–30.

34. Makdissi M. Sports related concussion – management in general practice. Aust Fam Physician 2010;39(1–2):12–7.

35. Luckhoff C, Starr M. Minor head injuries in children: an approach to management. Aust Fam Physician 2010;39(5):284–7.

36. McCrory P, et al. Consensus statement on concussion in sport—the 5th international conference on concussion in sport held in Berlin, October 2016 Br J Sports Med 2017;0:1–10. doi:10.1136/bjsports-2017-097699. Available at www.concussioinsport.gov.au. Accessed 20 November 2019.

37. McCrory P, Meeuwisse W, Dvorak J, et al. Consensus statement on concussion in sport-the 5 th international conference on concussion in sport held in Berlin, October 2016. Br J Sports Med 2017;51:838–47.

38. Browne GJ, Dimou S. Concussive head injury in children and adolescents. Aust Fam Physician 2016;45(7):470–6.

39. Easter JS, Bakes K, Dhaliwal J, et al. Comparison of PECARN, CATCH, and CHALICE rules for children with minor head injury: a prospective cohort study. Ann Emerg Med 2014;64(2):145–52.e5.

40. Davis GA, Anderson V, Babl FE, et al. What is the difference in concussion management in children as compared with adults? A systematic review. Br J Sports Med 2017;51:949–57.

41. Makdissi M, Davis G, McCrory P. Updated guidelines for the management of sports-related concussion in general practice. Aust Fam Physician 2014; 43(3):94–9.
42. Centers for Disease Control. Heads up concussion. Available at: https://www.cdc.gov/headsup/basics/concussion_recovery.html. Accessed 17 February 2019.
43. Rutgers University. Athletes should build neck strength to reduce concussion risk, researchers recommend. Science Daily. Available at: https://www.sciencedaily.com/releases/2019/01/190116110948.htm. Accessed January 16, 2019.
44. Haran HP, Bressan S, Oakley E, et al. On-field management and return-to-play in sports-related concussion in children: are children managed appropriately? J Sci Med Sport 2016;19(3):194–9.
45. Gunasekaran P, Hodge C, Perace A, et al. A review of concussion diagnosis and management in Australian professional sporting codes. Phys Sports Med 2019; 48(1):1–7.
46. Dellazizzo L, Demers S, Charbonney E, et al. Minimal PaO2 threshold after traumatic brain injury and clinical utility of a novel brain oxygenation ratio. J Neurosurg 2019;131:1639–47.
47. Joaquim A, Ghizoni E, Tedeschi H, et al. In: Fundamentals of Neurosurgery. A guide for clinicians and medical students. Cham, Switzerland: Springer; 2019. ISBN: 978-3-030-17648-8.
48. National Disability Insurance Scheme (NIDIS). Australian government. Available at: https://www.ndis.gov.au. Accessed October 16, 2019.
49. Zhu Z, Zhang W, Wu C. Energy conversion in woodpecker on successive pecking and its role on anti-shock protection of brain. China Technol Sci 2014;57:1269.

Use of Diaries in Intensive Care Unit Delirium Patients
German Nursing Perspectives

Peter Nydahl, RN, MScN, PhD[a],*, Teresa Deffner, PhD[b]

KEYWORDS

- Delirium • Diary • Intensive care unit • Post–intensive care syndrome • Coping

KEY POINTS

- Delirium is a common complication in critical care patients.
- Most delirious patients have frightening experiences and delusional memories but cannot remember the whole period.
- Diaries, written for critical care patients by staff and families and read by patients after critical illness, may help in coping with the experience of delirium and in understanding what happened.

Mr Smith[a] is 72 years old and lived at home with his beloved wife. He is proud father of 2 children and even prouder of his 2-year-old granddaughter. He is a retired truck driver and likes walking with his dog and gardening. Life left its marks, and he became obese (body mass index of 35) and developed chronic obstructive pulmonary disease and diabetes mellitus. Three days ago, he caught a cold and was coughing a lot. His wife was worried and told him to go to the doctor, but he declined. This morning, he is lying in bed, gasping for air. His wife called the ambulance. Mr Smith is admitted to the hospital with severe pneumonia. One day later, his condition worsened, he developed fever, delirium, requires supplemental oxygen, and during the day he developed an acute respiratory disease syndrome (ARDS). In the evening he is admitted on an intensive care unit (ICU), gasping for air, shouting, and frightened. During the night he is intubated and connected to a ventilator. For efficient

[a] Nursing Research, Department of Anaesthesiology and Intensive Care Medicine, University Hospital Schleswig-Holstein, Campus Kiel, Arnold-Heller-Str. 3, Haus V40, Kiel 24105, Germany;
[b] Department of Anesthesiology and Intensive Care Medicine, Jena University Hospital, Am Klinikum 1, 07743 Jena, Germany
* Corresponding author.
E-mail address: Peter.Nydahl@uksh.de
Twitter: @NydahlPeter (P.N.)

[a] The name is a pseudonym, and the diary entries are fictional, representing common entries.

therapy, he received high doses of analgesia, sedation and has a prone position in bed. Ms Smith is informed by the physician in charge. She is shocked and nearly collapsed.

POST–INTENSIVE CARE SYNDROME

Mr Smith has a critical illness and will spend some days on the ICU. He has a chance to survive, but what will that mean? It means that he and his wife will work on the consequences of critical illness probably for the next couple of years, maybe for the rest of their lives.[1,2] Survivors of severe critical illness, such as sepsis or ARDS, are at a high risk for post–intensive care syndrome (PICS).[3,4] This syndrome includes several consequences of critical illness, such as physical impairments (ICU-acquired weakness, impaired physical function, decreased pulmonary function, and so forth), cognitive impairments (impaired attention, memory deficits, reduced processing speed, and so forth), and psychological disorders, such as anxiety, depression, and posttraumatic stress disorder (PTSD). An estimated 25% of critical illness survivors experience PTSD, 34% depression, and 40% anxiety within the first 6 months after ICU discharge.[5–7] Risk factors are psychiatric history but also use of benzodiazepines and opiates during critical care and memories of frightening ICU experiences.[8] PICS can last for years.[9]

Family members and friends also can be affected by critical illness and are at risk for developing PICS–family.[10] The prevalence of long-term sequelae in family caregivers ranges from 4% to 94% for depression, 2% to 80% for anxiety, and 3% to 62% for PTSD. Common risk factors identified for adverse psychological outcomes include younger caregiver age, caregiver relationship to the patient, lower socioeconomic status, and female sex.[11]

INTENSIVE CARE UNIT DIARIES

How can patients and families be prevented from PICS? There are several options, such as early rehabilitation and mobilization, light or no sedation, delirium management, integration of families, and writing ICU diaries.[1,12,13] The basic idea of ICU diaries is simple: during critical illness, a diary is written for the patient by the staff and relatives so that the patient can read the diary afterward to fill in memory gaps and to cope with the experiences.[14] ICU diaries were developed in Scandinavia in the 1980s.[15] In Germany, diaries for ICU patients were unknown until 2008, according to a survey with a systematic screening of all 120 ICUs in 2 federal states of Germany, 23 nursing universities, and 19 experts.[16] Then, a network was created, delivering a Web site, newsletters, summaries of publications, lectures, templates, and other support. In 2014, another survey, including all 152 ICUs of the same 2 federal states and a further 69 clinicians, was conducted and found that 20% of the surveyed ICUs were using diaries.[17] Diaries are used worldwide today.[18] Diary entries are written in common language, addressed to the patient—"Dear Mr Smith, today I took care of you ..."—and authored by nurses, relatives, others.[19] Clinicians mostly write diaries to document what happened during critical illness, to explain possible frightening experiences, to prevent PTSD, to explain and reflect nursing and caring activities,[20,21] and to address the patient as person[22] (see example diary entries). Families mostly write diaries to keep the relationship with the patient, to communicate with the patient, and to cope with the situation[23] (see example diary entries).

Mr Smith's Diary, Entry #1

Dear Mr Smith,
Today you were admitted to the ICU. You suffer from a severe pneumonia. When you were transferred to us, you were coughing and gasping for air. You seemed to be panicked, shouting for your wife. I was holding your hand and trying to calm you, but your condition worsened. We decided to intubate you, connecting you to a ventilator, a kind of breathing machine. You are receiving sedation for sleeping. To help you understanding your experiences, we are writing this diary for you. We hope that it will help you to understand what happened.

—Nurse Betty, Oct. 10th

Structure and Use of Diaries

In general, diaries include a cover page with a picture, an instructional text with a how-to-write guide, information about the patient, and free pages for the diary. Sometimes diaries include a glossary, including pictures of the ICU equipment and staff, and some ICUs use photos of the patient but others do not.[18] Most often, ICU diaries are adapted to local culture and conditions. Hence, the structure and use of diaries are heterogenous,[24] as in Germany.[17]

Indication of Diaries

The original indications for using diaries were for patients on mechanical ventilation with an expected stay of more than 48 hours in an ICU.[14] Due to changes in sedation management and a broader use of diaries, today diaries also are used for all patients with probable disturbances in their consciousness, such as patients on mechanical ventilation or in delirium, coma, or deep sedation but also those in a palliative state.[18] Families of adult critical care patients and also parents may benefit from ICU diaries.[25,26] Contraindications are not known, but a diary would make no sense in patients with language restrictions, such as severe aphasia (but for the family). Foreign language might be not a problem because a team might provide a diary to the family or use translators.

Mr Smith's Diary, Entry #4

My dear,
I am standing at your bedside and cannot believe it. It happened so fast and now you are in critical care. The doctors and nurses are all very kind, they explained that thing with your lungs and why you require so many drugs and machines. I love you so and I hope that you will be healthy soon. We will manage this together, my dear. I love you.

Extent and Application in Germany

Indication and application of diaries are different aspects. In a survey in Germany in 2014, the authors found that starting a diary "depends on the nurse at the bedside."[17] There were a few ICUs with clear indications for starting a diary, but most times the responsible nurse initiated a diary or the head nurse suggested it. Writing diaries is a voluntary approach in Germany and the authors found no ICU team where 100% of staff joined writing. Some did not accept the idea, others did not like to write with pen and paper because of an unfavorable handwriting style or dyslexia, some felt time pressure, and others loved it. Diaries could be delivered in teams if approximately 50% of staff joined in writing; the diary-writing nurses became primary nurses of the patients with diaries, and a continuity in care and writing could be established. German nurses are writing diaries as part of a holistic care, not only caring the body of a patient but also serving the whole person, including the family. They are writing to do something good for the patient, to prevent PTSD, to fill in the memory gaps, and for other reasons.[17] In some German ICUs, the diaries are provided by psychologists, who often conduct follow-up care and evaluation with critical ill patients.[27]

Mr Smith's Diary, Entry #8

Dear Mr Smith,
You are on the fourth day in the ICU and the third day that I am taking care of you.
Your lungs are improving, and we are reducing your sleeping drugs. This morning,
when I called you by your name, you twinkled with your eyes. We are trying to
wean you from the ventilator, and you seem to be a little stressed. Maybe you
remember the situation when you came into the hospital? I am talking to you all
the time, explaining what is going on. You seem to calm a little bit. Your children
arrived and were talking to you. They hung up pictures of your dog and the grand-
child, and finally you opened your eyes. Welcome back, Mr Smith!
*   —Nurse Rodriguez, Oct. 14th*

Delirium

Approximately 40% of critical ill patients experience delirium and respiratory acute encephalopathy.[12,28] Delirium is characterized by disturbances in attention, perception, and cognition that cannot be explained by other neurologic disorders; an acute-onset; and a fluctuating course and is a consequence of a physical condition.[29] Delirium is seen as a result of predisposing factors, such as age, dementia, diabetes mellitus, and so forth; triggering factors, such as severe infection, stroke, hypoxemia, and so forth; and in combination with environmental factors, such as immobility, sleep disturbances, and so forth.[30] Consequences of delirium result in an increased risk for more complications, longer stay in hospital, dementia, mortality, and other complications.[29]

Delirious patients often experience frightening situations,[31] misunderstanding the situation, or hallucinations. They report an altered reality, disturbed sense of time, and existential fear of death: "You know, I'd wake up...well like somebody is holding your head underwater or strangulations was a major theme of the scary dreams I had."[31] Some experience frightening situations like being murdered or captured: "This happened in the hotel room where I was kept captive."[32] Delirious patients may experience intense feelings, such as fear ("Afraid, yes ... afraid and you do not understand why, you start to think how long I had to stay imprisoned"), frustration ("I was upset with myself because I could not catch what was happening"), or shame ("I was such a bad egg. I really feel guilty").[33] Approximately 80% of delirious patients are able to remember delirious episodes, but half not remembering the beginning and the other half not remembering the end[33]: "Now I realize that they were bad dreams. Up until 3 days ago, all that stuff actually happened to me ... Now I realize I was hallucinating."[34]

Mr Smith's Diary, Entry #11

Dear Mr Smith,
You are still at the ventilator, and sometimes you seem to be a little bit confused.
When I asked you, you wrote something about spiders and strange persons in the
room. You seemed to be scared and delirious. Unfortunately, this often happens
to critical care patients. We evaluated the reasons and we changed the central
venous line, and you are receiving new antibiotics.

Today, you were sitting the first time in a chair and this seemed to improve your cognition and condition. When your wife came in, she was so happy. She is sitting beside you, holding your hand. We all take care of you!
                                                                                    —*Nurse Betty, Oct. 16th*

Delirious patients have delusional, often frightening, memories, not knowing what is real or hallucinated, with intense stressed feelings that may lead to long-lasting disturbances and cognitive decline.[29] The evidence of delirium causing PTSD still is not clear and is conflicting.[35] It seems plausible that delirium is an indication for writing diaries. Nurses and psychologist providing diaries intend to close the memory gap, offer explanations for coping, explain interventions and examinations, assist as a base for understanding and developing meaning,[20,36,37] and also serve as a tool for relatives who might experience extremely stressful situations of witnessing a beloved one with delirium.[38,39]

Mr Smith's Diary, Entry #13

Dear Mr Smith,
Today was a busy day. You spent some hours in an examination in another department, and when you came back, you were sedated again. When you woke up, you became very agitated. You tried to pull out some of the life-saving tubes and you could not be calmed by words. For your own safety, we had to give you a calming, sedating drug and apply restraints on your body. You looked very frightened and I wonder what you were experiencing? I often told and repeated to you that you are in the hospital and safe, and that we all take care of you. Slowly, you seem to relax.
                                                                                    —*Nurse Betty, Oct. 17th*

Writing for Delirious Patients

The writing style for delirious patients is a little bit different from entries written to non-delirious patients. Although clinicians tend to describe their activities in cases of sedated patients, a patient's experience itself is more relevant during delirium. In any case, all statements made by the patient should be written down, even if they cannot be put together in a meaningful way (eg, individual spoken or written words or phrases). Ideally, these are framed by contextual information like movements of the patient, surrounding noises, or nursing activities. A detailed and hypothesizing description of patients' current mental condition also is important. All of these "fragments" can be significant for a patient later, because they are potential connecting points to existing factual or nonfactual memories, which patients often remember in detail.[40] The writing style during delirium thus focuses parallel to the medical treatment to the patient's perspective regarding his/her situation. Descriptions can be enriched by the nursing staff's interpretations of what the patient's behavior could be related to. In addition, and if possible, all visits of relatives should be entered in the diary.

Mr Smith's Diary, Entry #15

Dear Mr Smith,
Today I took care of you. You are still suffering from delirium and your state is fluctuating. In the morning you were withdrawn, sleepy and when you opened your eyes, you looked at the ceiling. When I spoke to you, you looked surprised, and then you drifted away. Some hours later, you became restless, gesturing, and were trying to communicate. Because of your breathing tube, you are not able to speak, but maybe you think that you are speaking loudly? I gave pen and paper to you, and you wrote "what is going on?" on the paper. I explained the situation to you, and it seemed to be hard for you to understand that you are in a hospital. A lot

of patients lose orientation, and maybe you perceive you would be somewhere else? Your wife will come soon, and I guess she will be the best person for you! I keep your written note in the diary—maybe it will help you some day to understand and explain your memories.

—Nurse Rodriguez, Oct. 19th

Function of Diary Entries

Detailed descriptions of patients' behavior and verbal statements as written diary entries can connect to patients' existing nonfactual memories. Diary entries show that patients' perceived reality does not coincide with factual events because medical treatments that tell an alternative story are described simultaneously. Confronted with these competing realities, patients can retrace the process of segregation between factual and nonfactual memories. In addition, the patient receives retrospective evidence for the support through and emotions of his/her relatives. Because the diary entries of relatives often contain expressions of love to the patient, they confirm social support, which is an important protective factor for preventing PTSD.[41] In addition to information from relatives, the diary is, after the ICU stay, initially the only source to thematically track a long period of unconsciousness or altered consciousness and, therefore, important for gaining a sense of coherence.[42,43] From a psychotraumatological perspective, the diary thus helps to retrospectively add another perspective to the patients' experience, which is essential for labeling a situation as potentially traumatic or not.[44]

So far, there is no evidence that a diary will help in in the special population of delirious patients to prevent or treat PTSD, anxiety, or depression or improve quality of life. As discussed previously, there is conflicting evidence for the benefit of diaries in delirious patients, but to the best of the authors' knowledge, no one has yet conducted a research specifically on this research question. Until then, the concept of diaries as a coping tool for delirious patients seems plausible.

Mr Smith's Diary, Entry #19

Hello Mr Smith,
Good news: your lungs improved, and we could remove the ventilator tube. Now you can breathe on your own and you can talk! You made it very fine! This morning you are much clearer in your mind. When I asked you for your orientation, you knew that you are in hospital, but not why. Again, I explained the situation. You told me of strange dreams, of being captured and a travel in a train. You tried to escape, but the train's staff kept you in a wagon. You said it would be very frightening and you were afraid of sleeping and in fear of this very vivid dreams. These experiences are common in delirium, and I explained this to you. I wonder how much of this experiences and dreams and information will be remembered, or will you be frightened of your memory? I asked you for your way of coping, and you said it will need time and small steps. God bless you on your way, Mr Smith!

—Nurse Betty, Oct. 21st

Handing Over the Diary

Handing over the ICU diary can trigger traumatic memories. Therefore, the handover and first reading are tied to requirements that should be considered. The patient should be fully awake and interested in his/her process of illness and recovery. The patient should feel confident and prepared for the possibility that he/she may experience intense emotions while reading. Presence of loved ones should provide emotional support and stability. Alternatively, professional psychosocial support can ensure emotional stability or recommend another time point for reading the diary if the patient is not well prepared. Of course, relatives also should feel able to accompany the patient during the first reading. If both patient and relatives have a burden of intense symptoms, reading should definitely be supervised by psychosocial professionals. There is no single recommendation for when to read the diary, and patients have different opinions about it.[45]

Mr Smith's Diary, Entry #22

Good morning Mr Smith,
Today, you will be discharged form our ICU. We organized a transport to a rehab facility and your wife is informed. She told us that she is expecting you there. We all hope that you will further improve your condition so that you can walk with your dog again and play with your grandchild. Maybe, you would like to continue writing this diary by yourself?
In case you have any questions about your stay on the ICU, please do not hesitate to call us, or even to come by and say "hello"! All the best to you!
—Nurse Rodriguez, Oct. 23rd

Promoting Recovery

As discussed previously, there is much heterogeneity in handing over diaries, and, of course, in rehabilitation.[24] In Scandinavia, diaries are handed over to the patients during a follow-up meeting 1 week or 2 weeks after discharge from the ICU; in some studies, diaries were handed over after 1 month or 3 months.[18] In Germany, diaries are handed over to the patient or relatives usually at the timepoint of discharge from the ICU, due to a high workload of nurses without time for a 1-hour follow-up talk.[17] Also, in Germany, most ICU patients are discharged to wards and afterward to rehabilitation facilities, where they spend 3 weeks or more with intense physical and psychological rehabilitation. Hence, follow-up meetings with former patients often are not necessary.[46] Nevertheless, the authors experienced some issues with reading and after-care of ICU patients. Some patients said that they needed up to 1 year until they felt able to read the diary. Avoidance is a symptom of PTSD; those who decline to read a diary may most benefit from it, but this is their own decision. The authors estimate the rate of nonresponders to the diary to be approximately 20%. This behavior may be one of several factors, decreasing the beneficial effects of diaries in studies and meta-analysis.[47,48] Despite these patients, the overall feedback for ICU diaries in Germany is overwhelming. Patients and families often come back to "their" ICU, with the diary in their hands and want to see Nurse Betty and others, who wrote such kind entries into the diary. Some national newspapers and even TV shows reported about ICU diaries, and the public knowledge of diaries as a tool for helping ICU patients and families is increasing. Anecdotally, some nurses for other ICUs told the authors that families started implementing diaries on their ICUs and invited the nurses to join in writing.

There is much work to do: electronic diaries versus handwritten diaries may be discussed[49,50]; diaries written exclusively by families in Germany evaluated[51]; the effect of diaries in stroke patients with temporary aphasia or in palliative patients evaluated; and more efforts made to extend the network and support implementation. ICU diaries should be part of a psychosocial care concept in the ICU that takes into account the needs of patients and relatives. The concept should be designed according to trauma-preventive aspects[52] and based on well-established psychosocial care structures for seriously ill patients (such as palliative medicine).[53] Although intensive care medicine can learn from multiprofessional psychosocial care in the neonatal ICU, oncology, and palliative medicine, the ICU diary as invention from intensive care nurses certainly can inspire other fields of inpatient and outpatient care.[54] In an ideal world, the diary of Mr Smith is written during the period of critical care and continued on ward, in the rehabilitation facility and finished at home.

Further information is available online: www.intensivtagebuch.de (German) and www.icu-diary.org.

CLINICS CARE POINTS

- There is evidence for the use of ICU diaries to reduce the risk of depression and improve quality of life in ICU patients after discharge, and also benefits for families.
- Delirium increases risks for cognitive decline, reduced quality of life, and others; the impact on PTSD is unclear. The benefit of diaries for patients in delirium is not researched, yet, but positive effects seem to be plausible.

DISCLOSURE

The authors have nothing to disclose.

REFERENCES

1. Mehlhorn J, Freytag A, Schmidt K, et al. Rehabilitation interventions for postintensive care syndrome: a systematic review. Crit Care Med 2014;42:1263–71.
2. Martin JB, Badeaux JE. Beyond the intensive care unit: posttraumatic stress disorder in critically ill patients. Crit Care Nurs Clin North Am 2018;30:333–42.
3. Needham DM, Davidson J, Cohen H, et al. Improving long-term outcomes after discharge from intensive care unit: report from a stakeholders' conference. Crit Care Med 2012;40:502–9.
4. Bryant SE, McNabb K. Postintensive care syndrome. Crit Care Nurs Clin North Am 2019;31:507–16.
5. Parker AM, Sricharoenchai T, Raparla S, et al. Posttraumatic stress disorder in critical illness survivors: a metaanalysis. Crit Care Med 2015;43:1121–9.
6. Nikayin S, Rabiee A, Hashem MD, et al. Anxiety symptoms in survivors of critical illness: a systematic review and meta-analysis. Gen Hosp Psychiatry 2016;43:23–9.
7. Rabiee A, Nikayin S, Hashem MD, et al. Depressive symptoms after critical illness: a systematic review and meta-analysis. Crit Care Med 2016;44:1744–53.
8. Bienvenu OJ, Gerstenblith TA. Posttraumatic stress disorder phenomena after critical illness. Crit Care Clin 2017;33:649–58.
9. Bienvenu OJ, Friedman LA, Colantuoni E, et al. Psychiatric symptoms after acute respiratory distress syndrome: a 5-year longitudinal study. Intensive Care Med 2018;44:38–47.
10. Davidson JE, Aslakson RA, Long AC, et al. Guidelines for family-centered care in the neonatal, pediatric, and adult ICU. Crit Care Med 2017;45:103–28.
11. Johnson CC, Suchyta MR, Darowski ES, et al. Psychological sequelae in family caregivers of critically Ill intensive care unit patients. A systematic review. Ann Am Thorac Soc 2019;16:894–909.
12. Devlin JW, Skrobik Y, Gelinas C, et al. Clinical practice guidelines for the prevention and management of pain, agitation/sedation, delirium, immobility, and sleep disruption in adult patients in the ICU. Crit Care Med 2018;46:e825–73.

13. Garrett KM. Best practices for managing pain, sedation, and delirium in the mechanically ventilated patient. Crit Care Nurs Clin North Am 2016;28:437–50.
14. Backman CG, Walther SM. Use of a personal diary written on the ICU during critical illness. Intensive Care Med 2001;27:426–9.
15. Egerod I, Risom SS, Thomsen T, et al. ICU-recovery in Scandinavia: a comparative study of intensive care follow-up in Denmark, Norway and Sweden. Intensive Crit Care Nurs 2013;29:103–11.
16. Nydahl P, Knueck D, Egerod I. The extend and application of patient diaries in German Intensive Care Units. Nurs Crit Care 2010;7:122–6.
17. Nydahl P, Knueck D, Egerod I. Extent and application of ICU diaries in Germany in 2014. Nurs Crit Care 2015;20:155–62.
18. Nydahl P, Egerod I, Hosey MM, et al. Report on the third International intensive care unit diary conference. Crit Care Nurse 2020;40:e18–25.
19. McCartney E. Intensive care unit patient diaries: a review evaluating implementation and feasibility. Crit Care Nurs Clin North Am 2020;32:313–26.
20. Egerod I, Schwartz-Nielsen KH, Hansen GM, et al. The extent and application of patient diaries in Danish ICUs in 2006. Nurs Crit Care 2007;12:159–67.
21. Roulin MJ, Spirig R. Developing a care program to better know the chronically critically ill. Intensive Crit Care Nurs 2006;22:355–61.
22. Parsons LC, Walters MA. Management strategies in the intensive care unit to improve psychosocial outcomes. Crit Care Nurs Clin North Am 2019;31:537–45.
23. Nielsen AH, Angel S. How diaries written for critically ill influence the relatives: a systematic review of the literature. Nurs Crit Care 2016;21:88–96.
24. Ullman AJ, Aitken LM, Rattray J, et al. Intensive care diaries to promote recovery for patients and families after critical illness: a Cochrane Systematic Review. Int J Nurs Stud 2015;52:1243–53.
25. Herrup EA, Wieczorek B, Kudchadkar SR. Feasibility and perceptions of PICU diaries. Pediatr Crit Care Med 2018;20(2):e83–90.
26. Nielsen AH, Angel S. Relatives perception of writing diaries for critically ill. A phenomenological hermeneutical study. Nurs Crit Care 2015;21(6):351–7.
27. Deffner T, Michels G, Nojack A, et al. Psychological care in the intensive care unit : task areas, responsibilities, requirements, and infrastructure. Med Klin Intensivmed Notfmed 2020;115:205–12 [in German].
28. Oldham MA, Holloway RG. Delirium disorder: integrating delirium and acute encephalopathy. Neurology 2020;95:173–8.
29. Oh ES, Fong TG, Hshieh TT, et al. Delirium in older persons: advances in diagnosis and treatment. JAMA 2017;318:1161–74.
30. Smith M, Meyfroidt G. Critical illness: the brain is always in the line of fire. Intensive Care Med 2017;43:870–3.
31. Gaete Ortega D, Papathanassoglou E, Norris CM. The lived experience of delirium in intensive care unit patients: a meta-ethnography. Aust Crit Care 2019;33(2):193–202.
32. Storli SL, Lind R. The meaning of follow-up in intensive care: patients' perspective. Scand J Caring Sci 2009;23:45–56.
33. Van Rompaey B, Van Hoof A, van Bogaert P, et al. The patient's perception of a delirium: a qualitative research in a Belgian intensive care unit. Intensive Crit Care Nurs 2016;32:66–74.
34. Guttormson JL. Releasing a lot of poisons from my mind": patients' delusional memories of intensive care. Heart Lung 2014;43:427–31.
35. Langan C, Sarode DP, Russ TC, et al. Psychiatric symptomatology after delirium: a systematic review. Psychogeriatrics 2017;17:327–35.

36. Storli SL, Lindseth A, Asplung K. "Being somewhere else'"*delusion or relevant experience? A phenomenological investigation into the meaning of lived experience from being in intensive care. Int J Qual Stud Health Well-being 2007;2: 144–59.
37. Thomas J, Bell E. Lost days–diaries for military intensive care patients. J R Nav Med Serv 2011;97:11–5.
38. Day J, Higgins I. Adult family member experiences during an older loved one's delirium: a narrative literature review. J Clin Nurs 2015;24:1447–56.
39. Mossello E, Lucchini F, Tesi F, et al. Family and healthcare staff's perception of delirium. Eur Geriatr Med 2020;11:95–103.
40. Darbyshire JL, Greig PR, Vollam S, et al. I can remember sort of vivid people...but to me they were plasticine." delusions on the intensive care unit: what do patients think is going on? PLoS One 2016;7:e0153775.
41. Guay S, Billette V, Marchand A. Exploring the links between posttraumatic stress disorder and social support: processes and potential research avenues. J Trauma Stress 2006;19:327–38.
42. Schäfer SK, Becker N, King L, et al. The relationship between sense of coherence and post-traumatic stress: a meta-analysis. Eur J Psychotraumatol 2019;10: 1562839.
43. Valsø Å, Rustøen T, Skogstad L, et al. Post-traumatic stress symptoms and sense of coherence in proximity to intensive care unit discharge. Nurs Crit Care 2020; 25:117–25.
44. Deffner T, Skupin H, Rauchfuß F. The war in my head: a psychotraumatological case report after a prolonged intensive care unit stay. Med Klin Intensivmed Notfmed 2020;115:372–9 [in German].
45. Egerod I, Bagger C. Patients' experiences of intensive care diaries–a focus group study. Intensive Crit Care Nurs 2010;26:278–87.
46. Peskett M, Gibb P. Developing and setting up a patient and relatives intensive care support group. Nurs Crit Care 2009;14:4–10.
47. Jones C, Backman C, Capuzzo M, et al. Intensive care diaries reduce new onset post traumatic stress disorder following critical illness: a randomised, controlled trial. Crit Care 2010;14:R168.
48. McIlroy PA, King RS, Garrouste-Orgeas M, et al. The effect of ICU diaries on psychological outcomes and quality of life of survivors of critical illness and their relatives: a systematic review and meta-analysis. Crit Care Med 2019;47:273–9.
49. Scruth EA, Oveisi N, Liu V. Innovation and technology: electronic intensive care unit diaries. AACN Adv Crit Care 2017;28:191–9.
50. Stone AA, Shiffman S, Schwartz JE, et al. Patient compliance with paper and electronic diaries. Control Clin Trials 2003;24:182–99.
51. Nielsen AH, Angel S, Egerod I, et al. The effect of diaries written by relatives for intensive care patients on posttraumatic stress (DRIP study): protocol for a randomized controlled trial and mixed methods study. BMC Nurs 2018;17:37.
52. Stuber ML, Schneider S, Kassam-Adams N, et al. The medical traumatic stress toolkit. CNS Spectr 2006;11:137–42.
53. Ferrell BR, Twaddle ML, Melnick A, et al. National consensus project clinical practice guidelines for quality palliative care guidelines, 4th edition. J Palliat Med 2018;21:1684–9.
54. Üzar-Özçetin YS, Trenoweth S, Clark LL, et al. Could therapeutic diaries support recovery in psychiatric intensive care? Br J Ment Health Nurs 2020;9:1–9.

Caring for Patients with Aneurysmal Subarachnoid Hemorrhage

Nursing Perspectives from the United Kingdom

Anne Preece, RN, RM*, Sally Young, RN

KEYWORDS

- Subarachnoid hemorrhage • Aneurysm • Vasospasm • Endovascular coiling
- Surgical clipping • Specialist nurse • Multidisciplinary team

KEY POINTS

- Aneurysmal subarachnoid hemorrhage continues to be a devastating condition.
- Treatment has advanced considerably over the last 25 years.
- Secondary complications remain a challenge to manage.
- The development of a robust pathway for treatment is crucial to improving care for the future.

INTRODUCTION

Spontaneous aneurysmal subarachnoid hemorrhage (aSAH) is a devastating condition that carries a high morbidity and mortality. It is estimated that there are approximately 100,000 strokes in the United Kingdom per annum. Of these, about 5% (8–12 per 100,000) are caused by aneurysmal rupture.[1] Approximately 600,000 patients are affected worldwide.[2,3]

aSAH carries a significant clinical and socioeconomic burden because it predominantly affects young people of working age.

On average, 30% of patients die before reaching hospital, and combined overall mortality and morbidity is estimated at about 50%, with 30% of survivors remaining dependent. This percentage equates to 3500 patients in the United Kingdom dying or being left with a severe disability every year. Secondary complications such as rebleed, hydrocephalus, delayed cerebral ischemia (DCI), sepsis, and cerebral infarction are the main causes of the disabilities[4]

Neurosciences Department, Queen Elizabeth Hospital, Mindelsohn Way, Edgbaston, Birmingham B15 2TH, UK
* Corresponding author.
E-mail address: Anne.Preece@uhb.nhs.uk

Crit Care Nurs Clin N Am 33 (2021) 47–59
https://doi.org/10.1016/j.cnc.2020.10.003
0899-5885/21/© 2020 Elsevier Inc. All rights reserved.

PATHOPHYSIOLOGY AND EPIDEMIOLOGY

aSAH is characterized by bleeding within the subarachnoid space in the brain, occurring secondary to the rupture of a cerebral aneurysm (**Fig. 1**). Presentation of aSAH is perhaps one of the most the well-recognized and characteristic in medical practice. In up to 80% of cases, a sudden-onset severe headache is the presenting factor. Typically, between 15% and 40% of patients describe a thunderclap headache or the worst headache of their life. This type of headache is often associated with nausea, vomiting, photophobia, impaired consciousness, and neck stiffness.[4]

Guidelines from the National Institute for Health and Care Excellence (NICE) state that aSAH should be considered in any patient presenting with sudden-onset, severe, and unusual headache, with or without any associated alteration in consciousness.[5]

Risk factors include smoking, hypertension, and consumption of excess alcohol. It is also more common in people with connective tissue disorders such as Ehlers-Danlos syndrome and in people with autosomal dominant polycystic kidney disease. The incidence is higher in first-degree relatives of patients with subarachnoid hemorrhage (SAH), especially if 2 first-degree relatives are affected.

The risk of rupture increases with age and is higher in women than men, at a ratio of approximately 3:2. In contrast with more common types of stroke, aSAH occurs at relatively young ages. Half of patients are less than 60 years old. The most common locations for aneurysms in order of incidence are anterior communicating artery, posterior communicating artery, basilar artery, and middle cerebral artery.[5]

RESEARCH AND CLINICAL TRIALS
International Subarachnoid Aneurysm Trial

The International Subarachnoid Aneurysm Trial (ISAT) was the first randomized trial of neurosurgical clipping compared with endovascular treatment of acute aSAH in the world and was set to dramatically change the treatment of this cohort of patients.

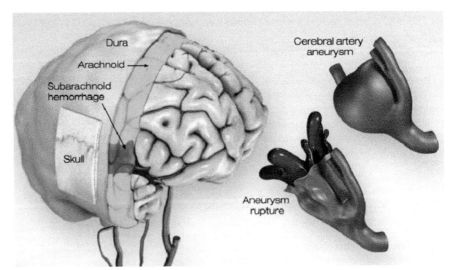

Fig. 1. An aneurysm. (Reprinted with permission https://www.stroke.org/en/about-stroke/types-of-stroke/hemorrhagic-strokes-bleeds/what-you-should-know-about-cerebral-aneurysms. © 2019 American Heart Association, Inc.)

The trial aimed to recruit 3000 patients over 4 years, recognizing that the clinical ramifications and impact on health care costs could be significant if substantial differences in patient outcomes were found.[6]

The principal aim of the study was to compare the safety and efficacy of an endovascular treatment policy of ruptured intracranial aneurysms with a conventional neurosurgical treatment policy in an eligible population.

The primary aims were to determine whether this treatment compared with neurosurgical clipping:

- Reduced the proportion of patients with a moderate or poor outcome (Modified Rankin Scale [mRS] 3 or worse) by 25% at 1 year
- Was as effective as surgery at preventing bleeding
- Results in a better quality of life
- Is more cost-effective
- Improves psychological outcome
- Long-term outcome over 5 years with specific reference to rebleed rates
- Long-term significance of angiographic results[6]

The principal investigators from Oxford, Molyneux and colleagues[3] published their findings in 2009. They had recruited 2143 patients with ruptured intracranial aneurysms, who were admitted to 42 neurosurgical centers, mainly in the United Kingdom and Europe. They were randomly assigned to neurosurgical clipping (n = 1070) or endovascular coiling (n = 1073). The primary outcome was death or dependence at 1 year (defined by an mRS of 3–6). Secondary outcomes included rebleeding from the treated aneurysm and risk of seizures.

The results showed that 250 (23.5%) of 1063 patients allocated to endovascular treatment had died or were dependent at 1 year, compared with 326 (30.9%) of 1055 patients allocated to neurosurgery, an absolute risk reduction of 7.4% (95% confidence interval, 3.6–11.2, P = .0001). The early survival advantage was maintained for up to 7 years and was significant (log rank P = .03). The risk of epilepsy was substantially lower in patients allocated to endovascular treatment, but the risk of late rebleeding was higher compared with neurosurgical clipping.[3,7,8]

This finding was supported in the Barrow Ruptured Aneurysm Trial (BRAT)[9] analysis, in which 362 patients had saccular aneurysms and were randomized equally to the clipping and the coiling cohorts (181 each). The primary outcome analysis was based on the assigned treatment group; poor outcome was defined as an mRS score greater than 2 and was independently adjudicated. The extent of aneurysm obliteration was adjudicated by a nontreating neuroradiologist.

From the 10 year follow-up, they concluded that there was no statistically significant difference in poor outcome (mRS score >2) or deaths between these 2 treatment arms. Of 178 clip-assigned patients with saccular aneurysms, 1 (<1%) crossed over to coiling, and 64 (36%) of the 178 coil-assigned patients crossed over to clipping. After the initial hospitalization, 2 of 241 (0.8%) clipped saccular aneurysms and 23 of 115 (20%) coiled saccular aneurysms required retreatment (P<.001). At the 10-year follow-up, 93% (50 out of 54) of the clipped aneurysms were completely obliterated, compared with only 22% (5 of 23) of the coiled aneurysms (P<.001). Two patients had documented rebleeding, both died, and both were in the assigned and treated coiled cohort (2 of 83); no patient in the clipped cohort (0 of 175) died (P = .04).

The conclusions were that there was no significant difference in clinical outcomes between the 2 assigned treatment groups as measured by mRS outcomes or deaths. Clinical outcomes in the patients with posterior circulation aneurysms were better in the coiling group at 1 year, but, after 1 year, this difference was no longer statistically significant. Rates of complete aneurysm obliteration and rates of retreatment favored patients who underwent clipping compared with those who underwent coiling.[9]

INVESTIGATIONS, TREATMENTS, AND COMPLICATIONS
Investigations

It is widely agreed that, on presentation, a noncontrast head computed tomography (CT) scan should be performed as soon as possible. If this is performed within 6 hours of onset of symptoms, the sensitivity in detecting SAH is close to 100%.[10–12]

If CT is nondiagnostic but there remains a strong suspicion of aSAH, then a lumbar puncture (LP) should be performed at least 12 hours after symptom onset. The LP should include a measurement of opening pressure, and a sample of cerebrospinal fluid (CSF) should be sent for (1) microscopy, culture, and sensitivity; (2) protein and glucose; and (3) spectrophotometry. A paired sample should also be sent for protein, bilirubin, and glucose[11]

When an LP is performed, the sample should also be sent for centrifugation to allow spectrophotometry for xanthochromia. Differential diagnosis for CSF xanthochromia includes traumatic SAH, hemorrhagic stroke (nonaneurysmal), hemorrhagic transformation of ischemic stroke, meningitis, encephalitis, and cerebral venous sinus thrombosis (with an increased opening pressure).

Sensitivity of xanthochromia on spectrophotometry declines over time, with a sensitivity of 70% at 3 weeks and 40% at 4 weeks after hemorrhage. If aSAH is confirmed on a plain CT head (or LP), an urgent CT angiogram (CTA) should be performed. A good-quality CTA detects greater than 95% of intracranial aneurysms. Cerebral angiography is still widely used in investigating aSAH; it is able to give reliable morphologic aneurysm anatomy. It is useful when deciding the best treatment options to secure an aneurysm[10,11]

Grading Systems

Common scoring systems that can grade the severity of hemorrhage include World Federation of Neurosurgical Societies (WFNS) score and the modified Fisher grading scale. Typically, WFNS criteria are applied once reversible causes of a low Glasgow Coma Scale (GCS) are excluded (eg, hydrocephalus, seizures).

Scoring systems indicate severity and can predict short-term and long-term outcomes. The scores consider GCS scoring and functional motor deficit. WFNS have shown predictability for functional outcomes in some studies compared with radiography findings alone[13] (**Table 1**).

The modified Fisher grading scale remains a strong predictor of complications such as rebleeding and need for retreatment, cerebral infarction, and DCI. It also correlates with mortality and poor functional outcome after hemorrhage[13] (**Table 2**).

Treatment

Clipping versus coiling
In 2013, the National Confidential Enquiry into Patient Outcome and Death (NCEPOD) recommended aSAH should be treated within 48 hours of ictus. Many centers adopt a target to treat within 24 hours from transfer and have local protocols in place. Patients with SAH should have rapid access to appropriate specialist care.[14]

The modality of treatment to secure the aneurysm (endovascular embolization or microsurgical clipping) should be determined following a multidisciplinary team (MDT) discussion between a neurosurgeon and an interventional radiologist. This decision should be based on a range of factors, including the patient's age, WFNS/modified Fisher grade, presence of large hematoma, location/anatomy of aneurysm

Table 1		
World Federation of Neurological Surgeons aneurysmal subarachnoid hemorrhage grading		
Grade	**GCS Score**	**Motor Deficit**
I	15	Absent
II	14–13	Absent
III	14–13	Present
IV	12–7	Present or absent
V	6–3	Present or absent

From Kundra S, Mahendra V, Gupta V, et al. Principles of neuroanesthesia in aneurysmal subarachnoid hemorrhage. J Anaesthesiol Clin Pharmacol. 2014;30(3):329; with permission.

(posterior or anterior circulation), overall size of aneurysm, and neck width. The presence of intracerebral hemorrhage and the need for possible clot evacuation should also be considered. The use of stents should be avoided if possible because the use of periprocedural dual-antiplatelet therapy increases the risk of complications.[3,7,9,14,15]

COMPLICATIONS
Rebleed

Rebleed is associated with a high mortality and, for survivors, there is poor prognosis for functional recovery. If a CTA or digital subtraction angiogram confirms the presence of an aneurysm and there is evidence of SAH on CT and LP, the aneurysm should be treated urgently in order to prevent rebleed. The risk of rebleed is approximately 4% in the first 24 hours, 20% within the first 2 weeks, and 50% within 6 months of initial hemorrhage[16–18]

Factors that can increase the risk of rebleed include delay in securing the aneurysm, worse neurologic status on admission (higher WFNS/Fisher grade), previous sentinel headache (previous severe headache that lasted for more than 1 hour and that did not lead to the diagnosis of aSAH, possibly representative of a minor leak from the

Table 2		
Modified Fisher score		
Modified Fisher Score	**CT Scan Findings**	**Risk for DCI (%)**
0	No SAH or IVH	0
1	Minimal thin SAH, no IVH	6
2	Minimal thin SAH, no IVH, with IVH in both lateral ventricles	16
3	Dense SAH, no IVH	35
4	Dense SAH, with IVH in both ventricles	34

Abbreviation: IVH, intraventricular hemorrhage.
From De Roxas RC, Barcelon EA, DioquinoMaligaso CP. Developing an evidence-based clinical algorithm for the assessment, diagnosis and management of acute subarachnoid hemorrhage: a review of literature. J Xiangya Med. 2017;2:24; with permission.

aneurysm), larger aneurysm size of more than 7 mm, and possibly a diastolic blood pressure higher than 160 mm hg. To reduce the risk of blood pressure spikes, a period of bed rest should be undertaken until the aneurysm has been secured.[18]

Between the time of ictus and treatment of the aneurysm, blood pressure should be controlled with a titratable antihypertensive agent to balance the risk of hypertension-related rebleeding and for the maintenance of cerebral perfusion pressure. It is widely acknowledged that hypertension should be monitored and controlled, but parameters are not well defined; however, managing a systolic blood pressure to less than 160 mm Hg is considered reasonable.[11]

It has been routine practice in neurosurgical units to prescribe supranormal blood pressure targets following coiling/clipping of aneurysms. Improvements in cerebral blood flow (CBF) have been noted but it has not been established whether targeting increased blood pressure by means of vasoactive agents reduces incidence of DCI and results in improved outcomes. Triple-H therapy (induced hypertension, hypervolemia, hemodilution) has been used for many years with insufficient evidence that CBF improves. Induced hypertension alone seems to be most promising in increasing CBF using noradrenaline or metaraminol.[19]

Hydrocephalus

Acute hydrocephalus is associated with neurologic impairment and increased mortality. It is common in patients following aSAH and occurs in up to 20% of patients within the first 3 days. The signs of acute hydrocephalus include deteriorating conscious level, poorly reacting pupils, and impaired gaze. Headache, vomiting, and blurred vision can also be signs. Noncontrast CT head can confirm diagnosis with demonstration of ventricular size.

Treatment with external ventricular drainage (EVD) may be lifesaving and can improve consciousness and responsiveness shortly after placement.[20,21]

CSF diversion with either short-term EVD or the placement of permanent shunts is a well-established practice for the management of hydrocephalus secondary to aSAH and is recommended by the European Stroke Organisation.[16]

Further studies have looked into the impact of CSF diversion on patients following aSAH. A meta-analysis undertaken by Qian and colleagues[21] analyzed studies comparing the outcome of patients who underwent any CSF diversion following aSAH versus those patients who did not undergo any form of CSF diversion. The meta-analysis concluded that the group that received CSF drainage had a lower incidence of vasospasm and infarction related to vasospasm after aSAH.[21]

It also concluded that the group that underwent CSF diversion experienced lower mortalities and improved functional outcomes, measured by a Glasgow Outcomes Scale higher than 3 or an mRS lower than 3. Only a proportion of patients with aSAH develop a shunt-dependent hydrocephalus.[21]

Delayed Cerebral Ischemia: Vasospasm

Symptomatic vasospasm is defined as the development of any new focal neurologic changes, or deterioration in conscious level, or both.

Cerebral vasospasm following aSAH is a well-recognized and potentially dangerous complication occurring most frequently 7 to 10 days following aneurysm rupture. This risk resolves after 21 days. It leads to a prolonged narrowing of cerebral arteries, restricting blood flow to the brain. The underlying pathophysiology is unclear. However, clinically significant vasospasm of cerebral arteries is thought to be related to spasmodic substances generated during the lysis of SAH clots.[19] Vasospasm causes symptomatic cerebral ischemia and infarction in approximately 20% to 30% of patients, which may result in long-term morbidity and mortality.[22]

It is one of the leading causes of morbidity and mortality following aSAH and is associated with clinically apparent DCI neurologic deficits in one-third of patients. Blood in the subarachnoid space is thought to trigger structural changes and biochemical alterations at the level of the vascular endothelium and smooth muscle.

There is strong evidence to suggest that oral nimodipine improves neurologic outcomes; by blocking calcium channels, it has a dilatory effect on arterial smooth muscle. NICE[23] recommended the use of oral nimodipine, 60 mg every 4 hours, to be continued for 21 days as a standard treatment following aSAH. Intravenous administration of calcium agonists is expensive and potentially hazardous in view of potential hypotensive effects and is therefore not recommended.

In the first 2 weeks following aneurysm occlusion, the prevalence of vasospasm measured by angiography approaches 70%.[24] Vasospasm can be detected with CTA, CT perfusion, MR perfusion, digital subtraction angiogram, or transcranial Doppler (TCD). These investigations should be analyzed alongside clinical examination. Euvolemia and a normal circulating blood volume should be maintained. If clinical vasospasm is detected, patients should initially be given an urgent fluid bolus to increase blood pressure and consideration should be given to initiating hypertensive therapy, unless preexisting hypertension or cardiac status precludes this.[10]

Neurosurgical units worldwide have variable access to resources for care, influencing protocols that guide management. There are benefits to certain modalities of investigation; for example, TCD has high accuracy for detecting vasospasm with a predominant benefit for middle cerebral artery vasospasm. It is noninvasive with no radiation dose and is minimally labor intensive. However, there are limitations, including operator dependence and lack of bone windows. For persistent or refractory vasospasm, transluminal cerebral angioplasty has been shown to effectively reverse vasospasm; however, there a very few studies that show long-term outcomes.[25]

Hyponatremia

Hyponatremia is a common electrolyte abnormality in patients following aSAH. The cause is not clearly understood, and the prevalence is thought to be up to 50%. Syndrome of inappropriate antidiuretic hormone secretion (SIADH) and acute glucocorticoid insufficiency are the main causes.[26] Acute hyponatremia is an emergency condition, because it leads to cerebral edema caused by passive osmotic movement of water from the hypotonic plasma to the hypertonic brain. SIADH is the retention of excessive water with normal renal function. Diagnosis is confirmed with:

Decreased serum osmolality (<275 mOsm/kg)
Euvolemia
Urine osmolality greater than 100 mOsm/kg
Urine sodium excretion greater than 40 mmol/L
Normal renal function
Hypovolemia (sodium level <135 mmol/L)

Eagles and colleagues[27] found that there was no clear link between hyponatremia and outcome but there was a more established link with the development of DCI. The causative factor seems to be the sodium level fluctuations that occur particularly with the aggressive use of hypertonic saline and that may cause more problems. More research is required, but, fundamentally, any irregularities in sodium levels should be treated promptly.[27]

FOLLOW-UP

Aneurysms treated by endovascular means usually necessitate standard 6-month and 2-year follow-up imaging after treatment or as per local protocols. The Cerebral Aneurysm Re-rupture after Treatment (CARAT)[20] study showed that recurrent aSAH was predicted by incomplete aneurysm obliteration and occurred at a median of 3 days after treatment but was rare after 1 year. Patients with adequately obliterated aneurysms after aSAH have a low risk of recurrent aSAH, although some do require retreatment. Patients with residual aneurysm or recurrence should be discussed in an MDT meeting with a view to discuss further treatment versus surveillance imaging. Longer-term surveillance imaging should be considered for those patients with residual aneurysms and should also be considered for the purpose of screening for de novo aneurysm formation in young patients or those with risk factors. Follow-up of aneurysms treated with surgical clipping usually consists of imaging to assess any residual aneurysm at an early time point. Again, longer-term follow-up and/or surveillance should be considered for young patients and/or those with risk factors for developing new aneurysms.[16]

The impact of aSAH can be varied and can include functional or cognitive symptoms or a combination of the two. A distinct feature of aSAH is the young age at which it can occur. Functional or cognitive symptoms can have an impact on day-to-day functioning and the ability to perform activities of daily living. There are often difficulties encountered with maintaining personal hygiene and these are concomitant with problems with visual memory, spatial function, and psychomotor function. Survivors commonly experience deficits with cognitive function, including memory, executive functioning, and language.[28,29]

Other difficulties experienced by survivors of aSAH include difficulty managing finances, shopping, and housekeeping. Many survivors have responsibilities with respect to work and family, and any of these symptoms can have an impact on how they live their lives. Buunk and colleagues[21] studied patients following SAH and concluded that only one-third of patients reported complete work resumption. Trial data from ISAT showed that 12% of patients require significant lifestyle change and 6.5% of patients were functionally dependent following aSAH.[3,28–30]

Al-Khindi and colleagues[24] studied the various impacts aSAH can have on patients. They found that, even in patients who make a good physical recovery, quality of life can be affected, as can life satisfaction. Anxiety, depression, fatigue, and a passive coping style are associated with reduced quality of life. The follow-up of these patients should include assessment of these factors and consideration of access to other services that may offer support. There should be access to rehabilitation services, psychological support, patient support groups, carer support, and consideration of referral to financial advice services.

MULTIDISCIPLINARY TEAM

aSAH frequently results in disabling psychological trauma, mental health difficulties, and cognitive impairments that can persist beyond the first year of discharge.[29] Salford Royal performed a long-term follow-up program using neuropsychology and specialist nurses to identify patients in need of neuropsychological intervention for ongoing problems that prevent return to work and a normal life.

An audit of patients revealed that 1 in 3 patients required referral. In the patients who completed the initial and final outcome measures, clinically and statistically significant improvements were seen. Results indicate effectiveness of joint neuropsychology and specialist nurse follow-up for patients with aSAH.[31]

The observed decline in intrusive thoughts and avoidance over time is consistent with that seen after life-threatening illness or trauma. The persistent reductions in independence and level of employment may in some cases reflect considered lifestyle adjustments rather than unwanted changes, but, in others, this indicates a need for focused rehabilitation.[30]

ROLE OF NEUROVASCULAR CLINICAL NURSE SPECIALISTS

A clinical nurse specialist (CNS) can act as a single point of contact for patients following aSAH. By following each patient's journey from admission to discharge, a CNS can offer a link between patients, relatives, and the clinical team. On discharge, with specialist knowledge they offer a link between the neurosurgical unit and community services and offer much-needed follow-up advice in order to help patients manage expectations regarding their recoveries. They can offer specialist knowledge on symptom management, possibly reducing attendance to general practitioners and reducing referrals back to the neurosurgical team.

Establishing links with rehabilitation units and support services in the wider community can have an impact on the recovery of patients. They can also advise regarding returning to driving or returning to work, assisting patients integrate back into their usual activities where possible or offering advice and referral to other services that may be able to offer additional support.[32]

DISCUSSION

In 2010, NCEPOD[33] commissioned a study to identify and rectify shortcomings in the care of patients with a confirmed diagnosis of aSAH in 27 secondary and tertiary units in England, Wales, and Northern Ireland. Previous studies concentrated on outcomes in patients admitted only to specialist units.

The information sought was related to organizational factors, initial assessment, referral pathways, quality of care, decision-making processes, interventions, follow-up, and delays as patients journeyed through secondary, tertiary, and rehabilitation care. A cohort of 687 patients aged more than 16 years presenting to secondary care following an aSAH during a 3-month period in 2011 was recruited. Questionnaires were sent to consultants in secondary and tertiary care with response rates of 82% and 79% respectively.

The principle findings were:

- Thirty-two percent of secondary care hospitals had no protocol for investigating the acute onset of headaches and 70% did not have formal transfer protocols.
- Twenty-two of the 27 neurosurgical units did not have a policy for defining the optimum timing of treatment of aSAH and 20 did not have a policy for preoperative management of these patients. Seventeen out of 27 units did not have interventional radiologists available 7 days a week.
- Almost 70% of patients in secondary care had not had a CT scan within an hour of admission.
- Forty-seven percent of patients were not prescribed nimodipine following diagnosis.
- Delays in referral occurred more frequently out of hours: 5.5% as opposed to less than 1% in hours.
- From Monday to Thursday, 72% of patients were treated within 24 hours, compared with 28% from Friday to Sunday. Only 8.5% of procedures were

performed by trainees under consultant supervision, highlighting the lack of opportunity for trainees to develop their skills.
- Ninety percent of hospitals could perform CT scans 24 h/d, 7 d wk.
- Following transfer to a neurosurgical unit, 95% of patients were admitted to an appropriate level of care and 86% were treated with endovascular intervention.
- Fifty-two percent of treated patients did not have the decision made in an MDT meeting.

Recommendations:
- The National Clinical Guidelines for Stroke[11] criteria for securing ruptured aneurysms within 48 hours should be met consistently and comprehensively.
- Formal networks of care should link all hospitals receiving were with aSAH to a designated regional neuroscience center.
- Standard protocols developed in secondary care should be adopted across formal networks from initial assessment and diagnosis through to rehabilitation.
- Relevant bodies should develop a nationally agreed and audited protocol for the management of aSAH in tertiary care from initial assessment through to rehabilitation.

In 2017, Zorman and colleagues[34] performed a survey was to assess how these recommendations are being followed across the United Kingdom and Ireland 17 years after ISAT and 6 years after the NCEPOD. An online survey consisting of 9 questions was electronically distributed to 32 neurosurgical units in the United Kingdom and Ireland. Only 9 (28%) units provide an interventional neuroradiology service 7 days a week, but all 32 (100%) units had established networks with other neuroradiology centers to provide aSAH treatment within 48 hours of ictus, assuming no delays in patient transfer. For patients with aSAH requiring neurosurgical clipping, 27 (84%) units provide (locally or through networks) aneurysm repair within 48 hours of ictus, whereas 5 (16%) units may breach this recommendation by keeping the patients with aSAH that present after 5 PM on Fridays and delaying their clipping to the subsequent Monday. Assuming no delays in patient transfer, 32 (100%) neurosurgical centers in the United Kingdom and Ireland meet the target of less than 48 hours from ictus to treatment for endovascular coiling and 27 (84%) units for neurosurgical clipping of aSAH.

Deshmuck and colleagues[35] studied the effect of weekend admissions on treatment and outcome. Weekend admissions were associated with poorer access to health care (ie, increased time from diagnostic scan to treatment and increased mortality). However, the excess in mortality could not be completely explained by weekend admission and it was suspected that other factors were at play that require further investigation.

FUTURE DIRECTIONS

Providing timely care for emergency patients with aSAH remains a challenge. Approximately 50% of admissions to neurosurgical units in the United Kingdom are emergencies, which comprise predominantly head injuries and aSAH. By the nature of the condition, this puts a strain on critical care beds, interventional radiology, specialist staffing, ward beds, and cognitive and physical rehabilitation.

The National Health Service England (NHSE) Clinical Reference Groups Neurosurgery Service Specification was published in 2019 and laid down the standard for neurosurgery in England.[36] In conjunction with the Getting it Right First Time (GIRFT) report,[37] the flow of patients through the system has clearly been identified as a major stumbling block for patient progress, with substantial regional variation. Length of stay in critical care varies greatly because of backup on the wards with patients waiting for rehabilitation. Management of elective patients has been shown to have a significant impact on the ability to accommodate emergencies because of patients waiting in inpatient beds for procedures instead of being admitted on the day of surgery, discharged promptly, or patients being converted to day patients. Recommendations from this report are now being taken forward by NHSE and the Neuroscience Transformational Group is the Expert Neuroscience Group. The aim is to develop a nontraumatic subarachnoid/intracerebral hemorrhage patient pathway. This pathway is due for publication 2021.

SUMMARY

The risk of rebleeding is greatest between 2 and 12 hours and is associated with increased risk of mortality and long-term dependent survival. Aneurysms should be secured within 48 hours of diagnosis. However, delays occur because of diagnosis and transfer of patients. Ninety-six hours is the current time it can take until treatment. There is a 30% mortality within 24 hours. Twelve percent of patients are misdiagnosed. Misdiagnosis can lead to a 4-fold increase in risk of morbidity and disability 1 year after presentation.

Nationally there is still great variability. The pathway is largely emergency; however, intervention for aSAH is generally not undertaken out of hours. There is national variation in access to interventional neuroradiologists and variability in the length of time patients spend in hospital after surgery.

The challenges for this service continue to be access to and sharing of diagnostic imaging, repatriation back to district general hospitals to continue treatment (eg, for rehabilitation), access to neurorehabilitation, and access to psychological and neurocognitive support.

CLINICS CARE POINTS

- The socio-economic burden of this condition cannot be underestimated
- In spite of the evidence timely treatment for this condition is still difficult to achieve
- Clinical Nurse Specialist input greatly improves the patient experience, providing invaluable support, ensuring appropriate treatment and referral and avoiding unnecessary hospital admissions

DISCLOSURE

The authors have nothing to disclose.

REFERENCES

1. State of the nation 2018: stroke Statistics. Available at: www.stroke.org.uk. Accessed 22/02/20.
2. Feigin VL, Lawes CMM, Bennett DA, et al. Worldwide Stroke Incidence and early case fatality reported in 56 population – based studies: a systematic review. Lancet Neurol 2009;8:355–69.
3. Molyneux AJ, Kerr RS, Birks J, et al. Rischmiller J for the ISAT Collaborators. Risk of recurrent subarachnoid haemorrhage, death, or dependence and haemorrhage and mortality ratios after clipping or coiling of an intracranial aneurysm

in the International Subarachnoid Aneurysm Trial (ISAT): long-term follow-up. Lancet Neurol 2009;8:427–33.

4. Maagaard M, Karissan WK, Ovesen C, et al. Interventions of altering blood pressure in people with aneurysmal subarachnoid haemorrhage. The Cochrane Collaboration. 2018. Available at: http://doi.org/10.1002/14651858.CD013096. Accessed December 12, 2019.

5. NICE. Guideline: subarachnoid haemorrhage caused by a ruptured aneurysm draft scope for consultation (22 August to 20 September 2018) Publication due Autumn 2020 2018. Available at: https://www.nice.org.uk/guidance/gid-ng10097/documents/draft-scope. Accessed February 2020, Accessed December 12, 2019.

6. Medical Research Council (MRC). International subarachnoid aneurysm trial (ISAT). Oxford, UK: protocolMedical Research Council of Great Britain; 1998.

7. Darsaut TE, Jack AS, Kerr RS. International subarachnoid aneurysm trial – ISAT Part II: study protocol for a randomized controlled trial. Trials 2013;14:156.

8. Kirkpatrick PJ, Kirollos RW, Higgins MNB. Lessons to be learnt from the international subarachnoid haemorrhage trial (ISAT). Br J Neurosurg 2003;17(1):5–7.

9. Spetzler R, MacDougall C, Zabramski J, et al. Ten-year analysis of saccular aneurysms in the Barrow ruptured aneurysm trial. J Neurosurg 2019;8:1–6.

10. American Heart Association & American Stroke Association. AHA/ASA, (2012) Guidelines for the Management of Aneurysmal Subarachnoid Haemorrhage: A Guideline for Healthcare Professionals.

11. American Association of Neuroscience Nursing. (2018) Nursing Care of the Patient with Aneurysmal Subarachnoid Haemorrhage. AANN Clinical Practice Guidelines.

12. Steiner T, Juvela S, Unterberg A, et al, European Stroke Organization. European Stroke Organization guidelines for the management of intracranial aneurysms and subarachnoid haemorrhage. Cerebrovasc Dis 2013;35(2):93–112.

13. Dengler NF, Sommerfeld J, Diesing D, et al. Prediction of cerebral infarction and patient outcome in aneurysmal subarachnoid hemorrhage: Comparison of new and established radiographic, clinical and combined scores. Eur J Neurol 2018;25(1):111–9.

14. National Institute for Health and Care Excellence. Interventional procedures guidance IPG106: coil Embolisation of ruptured intracranial aneurysms. London: DOH; 2005.

15. Lindgren A, Vergouwen MDI, Van der Schaaf, et al. Endovascular coiling vs neurosurgical clipping for people with aneurysmal subarachnoid haemorrhage. Cochrane Database Syst Rev 2018;(8):CD003085.

16. Claiboirne Johnson S, Dowd CF, Higashida RT, et al. American Heart Foundation. Stroke 2008;39(1).

17. Solanki C, Pandey P, Rao KV. Predictors of aneurysmal rebleed before definitive surgical or endovascular management. Acta Neurochir (Wien) 2016;158(6): 1037–44.

18. Salary M, Quigley MR, Wilberger JE Jr. Relation among aneurysm size, amount of subarachnoid blood, and clinical outcome. J Neurosurg 2007;107(1):13–7.

19. Van Haren F, Velloza P, Chan S, et al. Induced hypertension for preventing complications of delayed cerebral ischaemia in aneurysmal subarachnoid haemorrhage. 2017. Available at: https://doi.org/10.1002/14651858.CD012842. Accessed February 20, 2020.

20. Chen S, Luo J, Reis C, et al. Hydrocephalus after subarachnoid hemorrhage: pathophysiology, diagnosis, and treatment. Biomed Res Int 2017;2017:8584753.

21. Qian C, Yu X, Chen J, et al. Effect of the drainage of cerebrospinal fluid in patients with aneurismal subarachnoid hemorrhage: a metaanalysis. Medicine (Baltimore) 2016;95(41):e5140.
22. Adamczyk P, He S, Amar Ap, et al. Medical Management of Cerebral Vasospasm following Subarachnoid Haemorrhage: a review of current and emerging therapeutic interventions. Neurol Res Int 2013;462491, p. 1-10.
23. National Institute for Health and Care Excellence. Cochrane quality and productivity topics: calcium agonists for aneurysmal subarachnoid haemorrhage. London: DOH; 2017.
24. Al-Khindi T, Macdonald L, Schweizer TA. Cognitive and functional outcome after aneurysmal. Stroke J 2010;41:519–36.
25. Purkayasha S, Sorond F. Transcranial Doppler ultrasound: technique and Application. Semin Neurol 2012;32(04):411–20.
26. Hannon MJ, Behan LA, O'Brien MM, et al. Hyponatremia following mild/moderate subarachnoid hemorrhage is due to SIAD and glucocorticoid deficiency and not cerebral salt wasting. J Clin Endocrinol Metab 2014;99(10):291–8.
27. Eagles M, Tso M, Macdonald R. Significance of fluctuations in serum sodium levels following aneurysmal subarachnoid haemorrhage: an exploratory analysis. J Neurosurg 2019;131(2):336–656.
28. Buunk A,M, Spikman JM, Metzemaekers JDM, et al. Return to work after subarachnoid haemorrhage: the influence of cognitive deficits. PLoS One 2019. https://doi.org/10.1371/journal.pone.0220972.
29. Thompson. Cognitive and mental health difficulties following subarachnoid haemorrhage. Neuropsychol Rehabil 2011;21(1):92–102.
30. Powell J, Kitchen N, Heslin J, et al. Psychological Outcomes at 18 months after good neurological outcome from aneurysmal subarachnoid haemorrhage. J Neurol Neurosurg Psychiatry 2004;75(8):1119–24.
31. Khan A, Dulhanty L, Vail A, et al. Impact of specialist Neurovascular care in subarachnoid haemorrhage. Clin Neurol Neurosurg 2015;133:55–60.
32. Dulhanty H, Hulme S, Vail A, et al. The Self-reported needs of patients following subarachnoid haemorrhage (SAH). Disabil Rehabil 2019;48:1–7.
33. National Confidential Enquiry into Patient Outcome and Death. Managing the Flow? a review of the care received by patients who are diagnosed with an aneurysmal subarachnoid haemorrhage. London: NCEPOD; 2013.
34. Zorman MJ, Iorga R, Ma R, et al. Management of aneurysmal subarachnoid haemorrhage 17 years after the ISAT trial: a survey of current practice in the UK and Ireland. Br J Neurosurg 2017;17:1–4.
35. Deshmuckh H, Hinkley M, Dulhanty L, et al. Effect of weekend admissions on in-hospital mortality and functional outcomes for patients with aneurysmal subarachnoid haemorrhage. Acta Neurochir 2016;158:829–35.
36. NHSE neurosurgery service Specification. 2019. Available at: https://www.england.nhs.uk/publication/neurosurgery-adults/%20accessed20/02/20. Accessed February 2, 2020.
37. Phillips N. Cranial neurosurgery GIRFT programme national specialty. National Health Service England; 2018. Available at: www.GettingItRightFirstTime.co.uk. Accessed February 20, 2020.

Critical Care Nursing in India

Angela Gnanadurai, MSc (N), PhD(N)

KEYWORDS

- Critical care nursing • Self-driven empowerment model
- Integration of nursing education and nursing services • Dual responsibility

KEY POINTS

- Development of critical care nursing in India.
- Contribution of Society of Critical Care Medicine and Society of Critical Care Nursing in India in quality care of critically ill patients.
- Quality assurance in critical care in India.
- Integration of nursing education and nursing services as the model for critical care nursing in India.
- An experience is described of self-driven empowerment among critical care nurses through dual responsibility as part of the model implemented by the nursing services in a tertiary care center in India.

INTRODUCTION

Critical care nursing is an important part of the health care system in this technological health care world. The growth of critical care medicine and nursing in India is connected with how the economic changes in a country can lead to the evolution of a scientific subspecialty. Critical care in India has grown from a small body of professionals to a fully fledged active specialty. Globally, and with the focus on India, the growing geriatric population has started becoming a barrier to the much-needed critical care during emergencies. A systemic strategic plan is needed to overcome this barrier. The census in India has produced the findings listed in **Table 1**.[1,2]

The data related to critical care delivery in India, such as the number of beds, are unavailable because the registration of the intensive care unit (ICU) in a hospital is not a central process. It is not possible to get the exact number of ICU beds in India even now. The recent government statistics state that there is 1 government doctor for every 11,456 people. There are 535 medical colleges that teach 74,148 medical students and 4792 institutions that prepare 2,100,228 nurses each year,[3,4] but the population in India increases annually by 26 million. Thus, the available numbers are inadequate. There is a mismatch in the balance between the health care delivery

Jubilee Mission College of Nursing, Jubilee Mission Medical College and Research Institute, Kacheri, Thrissur, Kerala 680005, India
E-mail address: anggd07@gmail.com

Crit Care Nurs Clin N Am 33 (2021) 61–73
https://doi.org/10.1016/j.cnc.2020.10.004
0899-5885/21/© 2020 Elsevier Inc. All rights reserved.
ccnursing.theclinics.com

Table 1 Census in India	
Total population	1.24 billion
Gross national income per capita (PPP-initiated $)	3910
Life expectancy at birth (y)	Male: 64 Female: 68
Probability of dying aged <5 y	56 per 1000 live births
Probability of dying between 15–60 y old	Male: 242 Female: 160
Total expenditure on health as per capita (intl $)	157
Total expenditure on health (% of GDP)	4.1
Population living in urban areas (%)	31

Abbreviations: GDP, gross domestic product; intl, international; PPP, public-private partnership.
    Data from World Health Organization. Global health observatory. Available at: https://www. who.int/data/gho/data/countries/country-details/GHO/india?countryProfileId=e150dd37-4c59-4743-8c1d-e90c1d4a545f.

and the population and health care resources available. Thirty-one percent of the population, living in urban and semiurban areas get concentrated, high-quality health services. Corporate hospitals accommodate them along with other government health care facilities. Sixty-nine percent of the population, living in the rural areas, get only 15% of the resources, which are grossly unregulated, uncertified, and ill equipped.[2] This article discusses Critical care nurses society of India (CCNS), which has evolved significantly over the past decade. Types of critical care units, formation of the Indian Society of Critical Care Medicine (ISCCM) and Nursing, development of this specialty, and integration of nursing education and services toward the practice model of self-driven empowerment in critical care nursing are reviewed.

Fundamentals of Critical Care Nursing

Critical care nurses understand the function and disorders of every organ in the body. There are many parts of the body, hence critical care has many divisions, such as medical, surgical, neurology, cardiac, cardiothoracic, neonatology, trauma, pediatric, hepatogastroenterology, operating theater, and casualty. The specific care in each division varies and is highly specialized. Teaching other departments (divisions) and learning from them is an integral part of critical care nursing. The critical care unit develops a framework through which this learning is provided to all staff in the critical care units.

Communication for Safe Patient Care

Communication is vital in providing safe patient care. Patient-specific clinical information between health care team members needs to be accurate, complete, clear, and concise for continuation of care during each shift in the critical care units. The critical care nurses are trained to use a situation, background, assessment, and recommendation (SBAR) communication tool at all times. Awareness of situation, complete and correct information about the background, findings of specific and relevant assessment, and the recommendation for how to proceed in continuation of care helps in clinical-specific decision making. The SBAR communication tool can be practiced only if critical care nurses are updated in their knowledge of the disease condition, recent trends, protocols, and policies followed in the critical care unit.[5,6] Hence, it goes hand in hand with continuous in-service education, daily team conference, monthly review meetings on specific care, and availability of libraries (digital/books and journals) for references.

RECRUITMENT AND TRAINING OF CRITICAL CARE NURSES

Critical care nurses are recruited with care. Training, assessment, duty schedule pattern, and frequency of appraisal change from institution to institution. Recruitment procedure has inbuilt competency-based training for certain durations to cover the theory and practical assessments. After this, the nurses are placed in the respective departments. Until they are confirmed, they are posted under a preceptor/senior staff member. They are appraised every 3 months for a year, every 6 months for 2 years, and then their appointments are confirmed at the end of the third year. After confirmation, the appraisal is done every year. Twelve-hour shifts during the day are not as widely practiced as during night shifts. The following are the common duty schedules being practiced and found successful in critical care units in India. Plan A: 7.30 AM to 1.30 PM, 1.30 PM to 7.30 PM, 7.30 PM to 7.30 AM. Plan B: 7.00 AM to 4.00 PM, 3.30 PM to 11.30 PM, 11.30 PM to 7.30 AM

Educational Programs

Critical care nursing is physically, emotionally, and spiritually exhausting in India. The following critical care nursing programs are available.

1. The Indian Nursing Council (INC) along with state nursing councils has run 1-year Postgraduate Diploma in Critical Care Nursing programs since 1993.
2. The Postgraduate Nursing Program, one of the specialties under the Medical Surgical Nursing, Critical Care Nursing course, has been offered by INC through health care universities since 1995.
3. The Nurse Practitioner in Critical Care Nursing postgraduate residency program was launched in November 2017 by the government of India, through INC. This program is implemented in almost 24 colleges of nursing. The first batch of students were admitted in the year 2018 and they completed their course in 2020. The intention of the program in nursing was fulfilled and all of them have placed well in various institutions. The effectiveness of the program is yet to be measured.

Critical Care Nursing Society in India is vital to nurses. It was registered on 21 November 2011. It publishes the bimonthly *Journal of Critical Care Nursing*. It offers the Certificate Program in Critical Care Nursing (3 years), Fellowship in Critical Care Nursing (1 year), and Diploma in Critical Care Nursing (6 months).[7]

The Indian Society of Critical Care Medicine (ISCCM) was registered on the 9 October 1993. All the directors are trained from abroad. It laid down the course curriculum, identification process of training institutes, and their certification, as well as a well-structured exit examination. Initially a 1-year certificate course was started, which soon evolved into a 1-year diploma and a 2-year fellowship course. There is an enormous growth in the number of candidates registering for these courses over the last 3 years; there is also an increasing number of institutions offering these courses.[8]

Publications

The Critical Care Nursing Society publishes the *Journal of Critical Care Nursing*. The Society works hard to make it an index journal. The ISCCM has published the *Indian Journal of Critical Care Medicine* since 1996 and has been indexed in

MEDLINE since 2007. It is now published monthly and gets many articles from outside the Indian subcontinent. ISCCM has other publications, including a newsletter, *Critical Care Communications*; an ICU protocol book; an audio journal series podcast; and now a textbook, called the *ICU Book*. It has also published numerous guidelines (eg, on catheter-related bloodstream infections, management of tropical infections, end-of-life care, ICU planning and designing in India).[9,10] The critical care societies have taken adequate steps to collaborate with international experts through national and international conferences. The collaboration with specialists from around the world has done wonders to increase the level of scientific knowledge and professional standards and to introduce appropriate models of critical care to average ICU nurses, physicians, and doctors in India. Medical tourism has helped in promoting and advancing research in critical care medicine and nursing by bringing together leading experts in critical care, researchers, engineers, and scientists.

Integration of Nursing Education and Nursing Service in Critical Care Nursing

It has been found that integration of nursing education and the nursing services model in critical care nursing education has been effective in India. Faculty from the college of nursing take dual responsibility and their skills are fully used in the clinical area. Although more staff are needed in the college of nursing, this has contributed to filling the gap between nursing education and services, and, most importantly, has contributed to nursing research and helping to apply clinical research findings for better patient outcomes.

This unique blend of practitioners and teaching could be applied at primary, secondary, and tertiary levels of care. The availability of nurse managers in the clinical area who take dual responsibility with nursing education and nursing service makes an enormous difference to rendering quality nursing care to critically ill patients.

This model of nursing education is being practiced only in a few institutions. The INC took an important step by making a simple framework and requesting all the nursing education institutions integrate their nursing education and nursing services. It is encouraging that many institutions have decided to adopt the same model.

This model helps nurse managers to be part of policy making, advocacy, and quality assurance in nursing. This approach empowers leadership roles in nursing professionals and motivates the translation of plans into actions. This model is instrumental in building a positive and healthy work culture. Dual roles improves the standard of patient care as well as preparing competent, empathetic nurses with professional excellence in their fields.[11] **Figs. 1** and **2** explain the organizational pattern and the model for a quality environment for clinical learning through integration of nursing education and nursing services, respectively.

Quality Improvement in Critical Care Units

Hospitals and health care institutions undergo accreditation through national and international agencies. The widely accepted accreditation process through the government of India is via the National Accreditation Board for Hospitals (NABH).[12–14] NABH is an institutional member of the International Society for Quality in Health Care (ISQua).[15]

National Accreditation Board for Hospitals

Critical care units undergo an accreditation process along with the hospitals. The ISQua has accredited standards for hospitals developed by the National Accreditation Board for Hospitals and Health Care Providers (NABH) in India. The NABH is

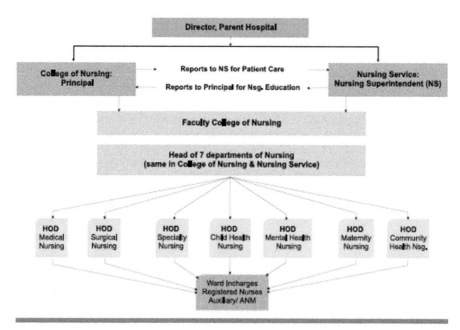

Fig. 1. Model organigram of integration of nursing education and nursing services. NS, nursing superintendent; ANM, Auxillary Nurse and Midwife; H.O.D., Head of the department.

committed to the improvement of quality of health care services in India for all strata of the population through various methodologies and tools to supplement the efforts of providers of health care services and the requirement of the health systems at various levels to improve efficiency and the predictability of health care outcomes.

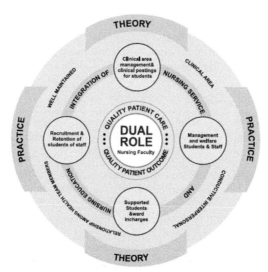

Fig. 2. Quality learning environment model for student nurses. This model depicts integration of nursing education and nursing service.

As many as 662 hospitals have taken full accreditation and many more have entry-level accreditation. This accreditation is valid for 3 years and can be renewed thereafter.[13,14]

Program for nursing excellence
The government of India under this scheme offers an accreditation program for nursing excellence. Nursing services are an integral part of the clinical services of any health care organization. The aim of nursing services is to provide comprehensive nursing care in terms of health promotion, prevention of diseases, and therapeutic nursing care to patients in hospital as well as to the community. The aim of nursing professionals is to provide safe, competent, and ethical nursing care with compassion, comfort, and collaboration with the patients, families, the community, and the clinical care team. The nursing profession is the cornerstone of any quality-related program in health care organization because most of the delivery and monitoring of health care is performed by them. Their knowledge, clinical judgment, skills, attitude, communication, and other soft skills make all the difference in the ultimate delivery of health care to patients. Standards are a prerequisite for the promotion of safe, effective, competent, and ethical nursing care. They help the individual registered nurses to evaluate the services being rendered by them and act as a catalyst for self-regulation and improvement. Nursing excellence standards have been framed with a view to laying down the guidelines for evaluating the nursing services being provided by a health care organization, thereby providing a platform for continued improvement.[16,17]

The standards are applicable to all the health care organizations irrespective of their size, role, specialty, and complexity. They serve as guidelines to nurse administrators and supervisors for supporting and facilitating safe, competent, and ethical nursing practices within their health care organizations. The nursing excellence standards have 7 chapters focusing on various professional, administrative, and governance aspects of nursing. There are 48 standards and 216 objective elements to accomplish. In future, many more institutions will come forward for obtaining nursing excellence and that in turn will take the quality of critical care nursing in India to the next level.[16]

The central government in India has made it mandatory for hospitals to be accredited and has made accreditation an eligibility criterion for registration of hospitals. Some of the states have taken a lot of effort to make it possible. This accreditation can improve the quality of critical care in India.

Critical Care Research in India

Original research in critical care medicine and nursing in India is limited. Through the following resources there is scope for the research culture in critical care to reach new heights in the near future:

- The contribution of critical care medicine and nursing societies and the Society of Indian Neuroscience Nurses (SINN) promotes research in critical care nursing.
- The syllabus for the introduction to nursing research in the BSc (N) and MSc (N) programs and research methodology in medical program will contribute to this improvement.
- Developing the research culture in every health care institution can encourage bedside nurses to conduct individual and group research.
- Critical care nurses need to be encouraged to take part in departmental research.[7,14]

Types of Intensive Care Units in India

Based on extent of involvement and supervision by critical care physicians and nurses, the ICUs function on several models:

- Open ICU model: patients are admitted under the care of an intensivist, family physician, surgeon, or any other primary attending physicians, with intensivists being available to provide their expertise via elective consultation.[18,19] The primary physician determines the need for ICU admission and discharge. The primary physician may not be aware of overall management plan, and this can result in conflicting orders and increased expense for patients.
- Closed intensive care unit model: patients admitted to the ICU are cared for by an intensivist-led team who make clinical decisions. This team has qualified intensive care physicians and nurses who provide quality care using ICU resources to patients, with better outcomes.
- Semiclosed intensive care unit model: the critical care team provides direct patient care in collaboration with a primary treating physician, although this physician is not part of the ICU team. Many surgical and cardiothoracic ICUs maintain this model.
- Mixed ICU model: the level of the intensivist varies. Both medical and surgical patients may be admitted in this unit.[18,19]

Quality Indicators in an Indian Intensive Care Unit

The quality of care in ICUs in developed countries is well described. In 2009, the ISCCM proposed quality control in Indian critical care units through benchmarks and standards.[20–23] This approach is feasible through electronic health records (EHRs).[24] In 2014, an ISCCM initiative addressed this issue through the Customized Health in Intensive Care Trainable Research and Analysis (CHITRA) tool.[25] It is expected that in 2020 there will be EHRs in 1.5% of hospitals to accurately calculate the quality indicators in ICUs in India.[24] Specific data for patients are captured and random checks are done in critical care units daily by the medical, nursing, and secretarial staff, who are formally trained.

As per ISCCM quality guidelines, the outcome measures from the quality indicators are collated.[26] Quality indicators are calculated using a standard formula that is provided in the electronic supplementary materials . First single-center report was published in 2014. The institution had an EHR stage 7. Ninety-eight percent of data were captured and were suitable for analysis. The findings were compared with the established benchmark data. The development of national benchmarks is yet to be established.[27]

Patients in the Critical Care Unit

According to ISCCM guidelines, the admission criteria are established. Facility for health insurance is not uniformly available. Awareness of health insurance is improved among lower and higher middle-class people. Self-paying patients account for 80.5%.[28] Hence, following any critical illness, the whole family can go into financial crisis.

Standardized Welfare Policy of Critical Care Nurses

The welfare policy for nurses in the government and private sectors in India differs. Hence the salary, leave policies, promotional avenues, patterns of salary revision and increments, leave facilities, and financial assistance for individual development, and an increment and recognition for additional qualification/specialization, are inadequate in most institutions. Hence, this has become a major factor discouraging professionally qualified and competent critical care nurses from remaining in India. Many migrate to other countries for better job opportunities and working environments. Constant steps are taken by the INC along with the government of India to change this situation and to treat the critical care nurses in India in the best possible way.

Practice Patterns in Critical Care Units in India

Although there is tremendous growth in intensive care medicine and nursing in India, few data are available on practice patterns in ICUs. Hence, it is not possible to reflect on the diverse spectrum of critical care illness, services, and practices in India. The availability of facilities in ICUs is not uniform across all ICUs. Most ICUs are open ICUs.[21,23,29] The critical care personnel with training are not associated with improved outcome because there are variations in the intensity and quality of training between the accredited ICUs. There is impairment in the monitoring of critically ill patients either because of unavailability or because of unused resources. End-of-life care practices need to be instituted in ICUs. Improvement is needed in many areas of critical care nursing in India.[30]

Patterns of Critical Care Delivery in the Indian Health Care System

The current practice of critical care in India is a matter of as much diversity as the country itself. Indian health care delivery includes 3 types of hospitals:

- Community hospitals are run by the government and at no cost to the patients. Because critical care needs a lot of technology and depends on finance, there is limited growth of critical care in these hospitals.
- Government medical college hospitals and districts and Thaluk hospitals: critical care facilities vary from state to state. Only small portion of these hospitals have properly equipped or staffed ICUs.
- Private tertiary care hospitals are managed by societies, trusts, or companies. They charge patients in proportion to their incomes. A small percentage of beds are allotted for free treatment. Eighty-five percent of patients are self-paying. ICUs in private tertiary care hospitals are well equipped and adequately staffed. Although major contributors of critical care to the country, they are expensive for patients.
- Small hospitals and nursing homes contribute 40% of hospital beds to the country. They cater to the lower-class and middle-class population. All patients are self-paying. These hospitals very rarely offer insurance. The need for critical care facilities is acknowledged and such facilities have yet to be fully developed.[30]

A MODEL INSTITUTION: QUALITY PROCESS THROUGH TRANSPARENCY, EDUCATION, AND SUPPORT

This author has 22 years of full-time working experience with dual responsibly in the institution. The experiences shared by the neurocritical care nurses are presented here. Empowering nurses at the bedside to implement quality initiatives has led to dramatic improvements in quality measures across the Christian Medical College, Vellore, Tamil Nadu, India (accredited with the National Assessment and Accreditation Council [NAAC] and the NABH, and has won nursing excellence awards for the past 2 decades). The details mentioned here are from the department of neuroscience nursing, where patients are most at risk. A high-quality clinical working environment for the nurses is provided through integration of nursing education and a nursing service model of practice. Nurses in supervisory and managerial roles have dual responsibilities.

Initiation of Quality Nursing Care

- The neurology wards and ICU set a goal of reducing the infection rate and it has worked. The neurointensive care department has a team of committed supervisors and critical care nurses. They innovatively plan and deliver the patient-centered care as a critical care unit team.
- As part of a multidisciplinary quality initiative, rounds were instituted twice a day, including an attending physician, quality improvement nurse, infection prevention, nurse manager, and the bedside nurse. The goal was to remove invasive lines and indwelling catheters from patients as soon as they became unnecessary and prevent the falls and pressure sores.
- At the same time, nurses perform meticulous screening of patients for any infection, as per the protocol, and are able to detect infections as early as possible as well as treating and preventing them.
- Critical care nurses are empowered to improve compliance with protocols in the ICU at all times.
- Every year, 6 to 8 clinical research projects are performed by critical care nurses. The patient outcomes are improving as the findings of the study are implemented.

Improving Nurses' Performance Through Transparency

Nurses' performance appraisals were carefully done, and the nurses were appreciated for their outstanding clinical performance. The nurse manager in neurology received an appreciation letter for her comprehensive report on a long-term patient in her ICU during the director's rounds. The letter stated that, "The culture here is 'not to be ministered unto, but to minister" to the work you do and be proud of it." I love working in a unit like this. We allow nurses to do exceptional work without interference and appreciate the ones who do. Nurses who need to improve their skills in specific areas are carefully identified, educated, coached, and supported without any bias. Nurses know exactly where they stand in their competency through constructive evaluations. It is a self-driven empowerment toward the quality process, she says. This transparency, awareness, and education have led to a reduction in procedural errors in the neonatal ICU (NICU). The nurse manager from the postoperative NICU stated that the regular feedback on individual nurses and where they need help to gain a sense of empowerment makes a huge difference.

Improving Nurses' Performance Through Education and Support

The nursing and medical leadership in the organization assist nurses to improve quality in other ways, such as encouraging and supporting nurses in pursuing higher studies. This support ultimately helps them move up the career ladder and translates to salary increases when they reach higher levels in their nursing careers.

- The provisions for attending national and international conferences are widely used by the nurses. Every year, 10 to 12 nurses from the Department of Neurosciences are sponsored to attend the annual conference of SINN and are encouraged to present scientific articles, posters, and models. These opportunities for education and support improve the exposure of critical care nurses and help them to develop networking with experts whom they meet in the conference as they learn more about their discipline.

- The benefit of this system is huge and rare in India. It improves evidence-based practice and comes back to the hospital to present new knowledge in ways that motivate nurses to improve their own practice. It sparks initiative and inspires neurocritical care nurses to begin research projects to be presented at future conferences. Everyone on this unit is a potential educator, learning, teaching, and working to improve quality. The critical care nurses here are leading the country by trying to set national benchmarks.
- The nurse manager in the neurology ward says that, "the experience of attending the annual neuro nursing conference is very enlightening. It gave me a new view of my practice and made me aware that we could improve the quality of research if more nurses were involved. My goal is to attend every national conference and encourage my colleagues to do so as well."
- The senior neurocritical care nurse says, "Everything we learn and share helps our practice. New nurses here will find people who open their arms and help. There is a welcoming environment, as well as support for updating the knowledge and an emphasis on conducting and publishing research to be presented nationally."
- The Professor and Head of the Department of Neuroscience Nursing says that, "The opportunity for higher education is intricately linked to quality improvement because of our focus on evidence-based best practices. Nurses begin to understand how we're driving quality at the uppermost part of the organization. The grand thing is that 8 of them from this department have been promoted to leadership roles."
- "Nursing has a voice at our hospital, and nurses play an important role in creating our processes," another senior nurse from ICU says. He acknowledges that nurses are supported through service awards, nomination of nurses for local and national awards, handwritten letters from senior leaders for outstanding performance, continuing education opportunities, and paid travel and attendance at conferences, to name just a few things done to encourage quality.

Other Supports

- Regular promotional avenues are available for nurses without any bias.
- The institution offers a free, high-quality health care facility for all the staff and students and 6 dependents of every staff member. The critical care nurse retention rates are the proof of the institution's success. In the future, nurses will have even more responsibility and autonomy. As the focus of health care reform moves toward keeping people healthy, nursing will become even more important and opportunities will abound for us to lead the way.

SUMMARY

Critical nursing is at the crossroads of development. The structure for quality practice has been developed but there is a long way to go. some areas So far, it is only working in some areas. Many forms of publicly or privately purchased health insurance provide limited coverage, and sometimes no coverage, for these services. The evidence that insurance makes a difference in health outcomes is well documented for preventive, screening, and chronic disease care.[28] There is lot of dynamism, opportunity, and development in this field. All efforts will make it possible to provide scientific and meaningful services to the multitude of critically ill patients in India. In addition, critical care nursing requires teamwork. It is important to create an environment where the opinions of all members of the critical care team are respected with the common goal of reducing ICU-related mortality in a cost-effective manner.

CLINICS CARE POINTS

- Based upon extensive review, survey and input of experts' ICUs were categorized in to three levels (Level I, Level II, Level III) suitable in Indian setting. Level III ICUs further divided into sub category A and B. Recommendations were grouped in to structure, equipment and services of ICU with consideration of variation in level of ICU of different category of hospitals.[31]

- An attempt has been made to propose a curricular structure / framework by INC towards preparation of Nurse Practitioner in Critical Care(NPCC)at MastersLevel.The special feature of this program is that it isa clinicalresidencyprogram emphasizing a strong clinical componentwith 20% of theoretical instruction including skill lab and 80% of clinical experience.Competency based training is the major approach and NP education is based on competencies adapted from International Council of Nurses (ICN,2005), and NONPF competencies(2012).[32]

- The ICU patients across the country show peculiar and distinct trends. During monsoon, 70-80% of patients are of infectious diseases (tropical febrile emergencies e.g. malaria, leptospirosis, dengue). Lifestyle related metabolic diseases and consequent critical situations are on the rise, e.g. diabetes, cirrhosis, uraemia. Consistent with the general demographic trends, 30-40% of patients in ICU are elderly, with inherent features of difficult weaning, prolonged stay and refractoriness to standard line of treatment.[33]

DISCLOSURE

The author has nothing to disclose.

REFERENCES

1. World population review- India. Available at: https://www.worldpopulationreview. com/. Accessed April 11, 2020.
2. Goel S. Doctor-population ratio in India, WHO recommendation. Available at: https://www.decanherald.com/bussiness/budget-2020/thedoctorpopulationratio. in.indian-is 14456against WHO-recommendation-800034.html. Accessed April 11, 2020.
3. Current statistics on medical education in India. Available at: http://www.mciin-dia.org>information-desk>for.students-tostudy-in–india. Accessed April 11, 2020.
4. Indian Nursing Council: statistics (Oct 2019), Distribution of Nursing Educational Institutions in India as on 31st Oct 2019. Available at: http://www. indiannursingcouncil.org/pdf/statistics-2019.pdf. Accessed March 20, 2020.
5. Müller M, Jürgens J, Redaèlli M, et al. Evidence based practice: impact of the communication and patient hand-off tool SBAR on patient safety: a systematic review. BMJ 2018;8(8):e022202.
6. World Health Organization. Conceptual framework for the international classification for patient safety. 2009. Available at: http://www.who.int/patientsafety/ taxonomy/icps_full_report.pdf. Accessed March 10, 2020.

7. Critical Care Nursing Society, India(CCNS). Available at: http://www. criticalcarenursingsociety.com. Accessed March 3, 2020.
8. Indian Society of Critical Care Medicine (ISCCM). Available at: http://www.isccm. org. Accessed March 3, 2020.
9. Praya S. ICUs worldwide: critical care in India. Crit Care 2002;6(6):479–80.
10. Nursing Reform, Paradigm Shift for a Bright Future, Aug 2016, Federation of Indian Chambers of Commerce and Industry (FICCI -Health Enterprise And Learning) (HEAL). Available at: FICCI_heal-report_final-27-08-2016.pdf. Accessed April 11, 2020
11. Chacko ST. Integration of nursing education and nursing services - dual role: a unique model. (Abstract of a paper presented in 10th conference of the Global Network of WHO Collaborating Centers for Nursing and Midwifery). 2018. Available at: http://www.esenfc.pt>event>event>abstracts>exportAbstractPDF. Accessed April 20, 2020.
12. Write JR Jr. The American College of Surgeons, minimum standards for Hospitals, and the provision of High quality laboratory services. Arch Pathol Lab Med 2017; 141:704–17.
13. The Joint Commission –Hospital Accreditation (JCAH). Available at: http://www. jointcommission.org/accreditiation/hospital.aspr. Accessed March 17, 2020.
14. National Assessment and Accreditation Council (NAAC). Available at: http://www. NAAC.gov. Accessed April 3, 2020.
15. The International Society for Quality in Health Care : ISQua. Available at: http:// www.isqua.org. Accessed April 3, 2020.
16. Nursing excellence –NABH. Available at: http://nabh.co/NURSINGEXCELLENCE. aspx. Accessed April 3, 2020.
17. Shankar R. Health Ministry launches " Nurse practitioner in critical care nursing , to meet the needs of tertiary health care services. 2015. Available at: http://www. pharmabiz.com/NewsDetails.aspx?aid=91763&sid=1. Accessed April 11, 2020.
18. Prayag S. Critical care in India : progress over two decades. ICU Management & Practice 2014;14(2). Available at: http://healthmanagement.org/c/icu/issuearticle/ critical-care-in-india-progress-over-two-decades.
19. Chowdhury D, Duggal AK. Intensive Care Unit Models-Do you want them to be open or closed? A critical review. Neurol India 2017;65(1):39–45. Available at: http://neurologyindia.com/text.asp?2017/65/1/39/198205. Accessed March 3, 2020.
20. Ray B, Samaddar DD, Todi SK, et al. Quality indicators for ICU: ISCCM guidelines for ICU in India. Indian J Crit Care Med 2009;13(4):173–206. Available at: http:// www.ncbi.nim.nih.gov/pmc/articles/PMC 2856147/. Accessed March 31, 2020.
21. Kiran KG, Bhuvana K, Sampath SR. Evaluation of quality indicators in an Indian intensive care units. Indian J Crit Care Med 2017;21(12):841–6.
22. Peter JV, Prithwis B, Dhuruva C, et al. Critical care quality upgradation enabled by Space Technology (QUEST), Guidelines committee. Indian Soc Crit Care Med 2017.
23. Delis H, Christaki K, Healy B, et al. Moving beyond quality control in diagnostic radiology and the role of the clinically qualified medical physicist. Phys Med 2017;41:104–8.
24. Sharma M, Aggarval H. EHR adoption in India: potential and the challenges. Indian J Sci Technol 2016;9(34):1–7.
25. CHITRA-customized, health care in intensive care, trainable research and analysis tool. Available at: http://www.isccm.org/chitra.aspx. Accessed March 20, 2020.

26. Divatia JV, Amin PR, Ramakrishnan N, et al. Intensive care in India: the Indian Intensive care case Mix and practice pattern study. Indian J Crit Care Med 2016;20(4):216–25.
27. Valentin A, Ferdinande P, ESICM Working Group on Quality Improvement. Recommendations on basic requirements for intensive care units: structural and organizational aspects. Intensive Care Med 2011;37(10):1575–87.
28. Swift EK. Institute of Medicine (US), Committee on Guidance for the National Health Care Disparities Report. Washington (DC): National Academics Press; 2002.
29. Plost G, Nelson DP. Empowering Critical Care Nurses to improve compliance with protocols in the intensive care unit. Am J Crit Care 2007;16:153–7.
30. Park JE, Park K. Park's Text book of preventive and social Medicine. 25th edition. Jabalpur (India): Banarsidas Bhanot; 2019.
31. Narendra R, Kapil GZ, Subhal BD, et al. Indian Society of Critical Care Medicine Experts Committee Consensus Statement on ICU Planning and Designing, 2020. Indian J Crit Care Med 2020 Jan;24(Suppl 1):S43–60. https://doi.org/10.5005/jp-journals-10071-G23185. Available at: https://www.ncbi.nlm.nih.gov/pmc/articles/PMC7085818/.
32. Indian Nursing Council, Nurse Practitioner in Critical care (Post Graduate –Residency Program) Available at: https://main.mohfw.gov.in/sites/default/files/57996154451447054846_0.pdf. Accessed November 12, 2020.
33. Yeolekar ME, Mehta S. ICU Care in India - Status and Challenges. The Journal of the Association of Physicians of India 2008;56:221–2. Available at. https://www.researchgate.net/publication/23170114_ICU_care_in_India_-_Status_and_challenges. Accessed November 12, 2020.

Critical Care Nursing in the Philippines

Historical Past, Current Practices, and Future Directions

Rudolf Cymorr Kirby P. Martinez, PhD, MA, RN[a,b,*],
Maria Isabelita C. Rogado, MA, RN[a,c],
Diana Jean F. Serondo, RN, SCRN, NVRN-BC[c],
Gil P. Soriano, MHPEd, RN[b,d], Karen Czarina S. Ilano, RN, SCRN[c]

KEYWORDS

- Critical care nursing • End of life and palliative care • Family involvement
- Pain management • Patient rehabilitation
- Interprofessional communication and collaboration • Quality and safety • Philippines

KEY POINTS

- The field of critical care nursing is widely recognized as a nursing specialty; however, there is no standardized national certification program for critical care nursing in the Philippines.
- The patient admitted in the intensive care unit (ICU) requires complex care and needs technologically advanced monitoring and resources; however, this has become a challenge in the Philippines because of insufficient national and local health funding and the prevailing health care financing system.
- There is a need to increase on the competencies of critical care nurses pertaining to pain and delirium management, provision of palliative and end-of-life care, communication, and interprofessional collaboration.
- Despite the central roles that critical care nurses play within the ICU, their active participation during medical/interprofessional rounds or patient case analysis is still lacking.

[a] Graduate School of Nursing, Arellano University Juan Sumulong Campus, 2600 Legarda St, Sampaloc, Manila 1008, Philippines; [b] College of Nursing, San Beda University, 638 Mendiola St., San Miguel, Manila 1005, Philippines; [c] Critical Care Nurses Association of the Philippines, Inc., 3rd floor, Edificio Enriqueta, 422 NS Amoranto St. Corner D. Tuazon St., Quezon City 1114, Philippines; [d] Graduate School, Wesleyan University- Philippines, Mabini Extension, Cabanatuan City, Nueva Ecija 3100, Philippines
* Corresponding author. College of Nursing, San Beda University, 638 Mendiola St., San Miguel, Manila, Philippines, 1005.
E-mail address: rmartinez@sanbeda.edu.ph

Crit Care Nurs Clin N Am 33 (2021) 75–87
https://doi.org/10.1016/j.cnc.2020.11.001
0899-5885/21/© 2020 Elsevier Inc. All rights reserved.

BRIEF HISTORICAL BACKGROUND

Critical care as a specialty practice in the Philippines was strengthened in the early 1970s. This was the time when then First Lady Imelda R. Marcos spoke about eradicating the country's top 3 killers (heart disease) by harnessing the advances of medical science. This was realized when the Philippine Heart Center (PHC) for Asia was inaugurated on February 14, 1975, with the goal of serving not only the Philippines but the entire Asian region.[1]

The beginning of this state-of-the-art PHC paved the way to strengthen not only the medical practice of cardiology but also the specialization in critical care. Soon after, specialty tertiary hospitals, like the National Kidney and Transplant Institute and Lung Center of the Philippines, were built, further enhancing the practice of critical care in the Philippines.

To complement the practice of critical care medicine, nurses working in the critical care units were trained initially with orientation, on-the-job, and *preceptorial* education. In approximately 1977, the PHC Nursing Service, Division of Nursing Education, crafted a 2-month postgraduate curriculum in critical care nursing designed to provide nurses with the concepts of critical care practice, such as cardiac monitoring, hemodynamics, mechanical ventilation, arterial blood gas interpretation, nutritional support, and Basic and Advanced Cardiac Life Support, among others. Although the original 2-month course was focused on cardiovascular pathologies, the integrated concepts of critical care were adapted by its trainees to enhance the critical care practice in their respective hospitals.

In February 1977, nurses from different hospitals, such as PHC, Philippine General Hospital, National Orthopedic Hospital, and Cardinal Santos Medical Center, represented by Amelia Baldovino-Lopez (founding president, Critical Care Nurses Association of the Philippines, Inc. [CCNAPI]), Deogracia M. Valderrama, Eufemia Rueda, and Ester Romano, convened to organize the CCNAPI. The CCNAPI has become instrumental in assisting the hospitals outside metropolitan areas to set up their own critical care units and has helped educate the nurses by providing various training programs relevant to critical care practice.

Currently, critical care nursing is practiced as one of the recognized nursing specialties that uses the nursing process to deal with potential and actual life-threatening conditions requiring organ support and invasive monitoring. It focuses on restorative, curative, rehabilitative, maintainable, or palliative care, based on identified patient needs, in a challenging and fast-paced environment.[2,3] The practice of critical care nursing in the Philippines involves a multidisciplinary, interprofessional, and a holistic patient-centered approach given in a timely manner.

CURRENT PRACTICE
The Critical Care Nurse

Critical care nurses in the Philippines are registered nurses trained and qualified to practice critical care nursing. They carry out interventions and coordinate patient care activities to address life-threatening situations that will meet patient's biological, psychological, cultural, and spiritual needs.[2] Within the current system, most critical care nurses have previous experience in the general ward before their exposure to the critical care setup.

Training for nurses who desire to practice in the critical care setting are usually provided by the nurses' respective institutions where the training curriculum is designed by their respective training offices or is collaboratively done with a recognized specialty organization, such as CCNAPI. The training usually includes a combination of didactic (lectures, seminars, orientations) and hands-on clinical components (preceptorship, mentoring).

Certification in critical care nursing indicates that the nurse has mastered the skills and knowledge base necessary to effectively care for acutely ill patients. Currently, there is no national certification for critical care nurses in the Philippines. Standards are in the process of being implemented in the Philippines.

Health Care Financing and Intensive Care Unit Capacity

Health care in the Philippines is mostly institution-based given through either public or private medical institutions. Metropolitan areas like Metro Manila, have a higher number of medical institutions compared with nonmetropolitan areas. Funding for hospitalization is paid by the national health insurance program managed by PhilHealth, private health insurance (PHI), out-of-pocket payments, or a combination of these. PhilHealth covers private and public hospitals with 30% to 60% of hospitalization cost; 50% to 70% for public medical institutions, and only 30% or less for some private medical facilities.[4] The rest are taken on by the patient either through PHI or out of their own pocket. These private PHIs mostly cater to selected private medical institutions and some public hospitals as well. Hospitalization in private hospitals arguably costs more than public hospitals and is mostly accessible only to those who can afford the out-of-pocket expenses. Patients declared as medically indigent are channeled to other sources of financing, and in some cases, fully accommodated by the government hospitals, with little to no financial burden to the patient and their family.

Most government hospitals rely on government funding, either through the central government or their respective local government units. Funding from the central government is relatively less affected by politics compared with their local government counterparts. To augment their funds, some government hospitals have been converted to government-owned and controlled corporations, allowing them to conduct commercial and noncommercial activities, such as allowing the patient the choice to be admitted either as a paying patient or a regular patient.[5]

The hospital's classification is reflected in the organization of its departments or attached intensive care units (ICUs). All hospitals in the Philippines are classified according to their service capability: level 1 hospitals have an average of 41-bed capacity, level 2 hospitals have 97, and level 3 hospitals have 318 average bed capacity.[4] Within this system, hospitals with higher level of classification can accommodate patients with more complex needs, and it is implied that they have more advanced technologies compared with those with lower level of classifications. The study done by Phua and colleagues[6] reported that there are a total of 2315 critical care beds among the 450 ICUs surveyed in the Philippines, with an additional 20 Intermediate Care Unit (IMCU) beds in 2 IMCUs, which roughly translates to 2.2 critical care beds available per current 100,000 population. Most ICUs are running near or on their limit even before the surge of cases brought about by the coronavirus disease 2019 (Covid-19) pandemic, which stresses and overwhelms an already overrun system even more.[7] With the current system, some patients requiring ICU admission are denied because of the unavailability of beds, forcing some of them to prolong their stay in the emergency department (ED), be admitted to a regular room modified to assist in their needs, or seek treatment elsewhere.

The Milieu of the Intensive Care Unit

Although there are IMCUs, often termed as intermediate care units or "step-down" units, most critical care nurses in the Philippines work in the ICU. These ICUs can be categorized according to age groups (neonatal, pediatric, adult) or medical specialties (surgical, cardiovascular, neurocritical, etc.).[6,8]

Patients referred to the ICU are those with potential or established organ dysfunction needing focused care and treatment. A patient may be admitted to the ICU via ED admission, transfer from the general ward, transfer from another hospital, or from a special or complex operation such as heart surgeries. Admission to the ICU is decided by the case of the patient, the availability of beds, the attending physician and critical care physician's collaborative management, and sometimes the demands of the patient's family who will shoulder the hospital expenses. There are instances wherein moribund patients, whose clinical outcomes may not be improved by ICU management, are still admitted to the ICU so long as there is an availability of beds and is done with the approval of the patient's attending physicians and their family. Patients admitted in the ICU are generally classified using varied patient care acuity tools depending on institutional preference.

Operation within these ICUs can be classified as open, closed, or a combination of both. In an open system, admission and patient management is the primary and sole responsibility of the attending physicians. Other physicians, such as the intensivist or critical care specialist provides advice only on the patient's management. The attending physician has the sole prerogative on the direction of the patient's management. Under the closed system, the intensivist or critical care specialist provides the decision on patient management. Once referral is done by the previous attending or admitting physician, the intensivist or critical care specialist will take over patient management.[2]

Regardless of the type of operation, a team of critical care nurses is always present to provide direct patient care as part of the multidisciplinary team. Critical care nurses are usually led clinically by a charge nurse and administratively by a head nurse. Although each critical care nurse works independently as they work under primary nursing, the charge nurse provides bedside clinical support if needed, whereas the head nurse answers for administrative concerns. Patient assignment and staffing are collaboratively done by both the charge and head nurses. At times, the charge and the head nurses are the same person, as many ICUs have concerns with low staffing. The decreased number of critical care nurses working in the ICU is attributed to the high attrition rate, as many will resign to seek greener pasture abroad, and to the low uptake of new critical care nurses, as most systems allow only those with bedside experience to be trained in the ICU setup, compounded by the fact that the application for any nursing post is generally low.

Staffing in the ICU is generally based on the availability of limited critical care nurses rather than the patient's acuity of care. The ideal ratio of 1 nurse to 1 to 3 patients in the ICU[2,9] is achieved only if there is sufficient staff available on the floor. Because the ICU is considered as a highly specialized unit, there is difficulty of "floating" nurses from other wards when staffing is low, thus patient assignment among critical care nurses present within the shift will be higher than the ideal ratio. With these, the possibility of an overtime duty among critical care nurses is a daily reality. Shifts may vary from an 8-hour to 12-hour duty per day with a required minimum of 40 hours per week for a full-time post. Almost all critical care nurses work full-time. This less-than-ideal staffing setup significantly contributes to the perceived unfavorable and frustrating work environment among critical care nurses along with their heavy workload, perceived lack of mentorship, and standardized national training guidelines.[10]

Patient assignments are generally given during shift handover, often referred to in the Philippines as "endorsement." Although the process of handover varies from different institutions, the same goal of a complete handover of care from the outgoing to the incoming shift is still attained. The handover among physicians and among nurses happens at different times because of the variation in their shifting schedules. Tools used during handover vary across different ICU units, but are consistent among related institutions, such as hospital conglomerates.

Patients admitted in the ICU needing transport to and from a different part of the hospital or from another medical institution are accompanied by at least 1 physician, 1 nurse trained in critical care, and various support personnel, such as nursing aide, respiratory therapist, and other allied health care personnel depending on the need and equipment attached to the patient during transport. Interinstitutional patient transfer, often referred to as "conduction," is mostly done if the needed diagnostics are not present in the institution, as is often the case in government hospitals, or if the patient decides to change hospitals for better care, or because of lack of funding. During these interinstitutional transfers, a medical technician and/or a paramedic may be present depending on the circumstances. Although transport policies and guidelines markedly vary within medical institutions, the role of critical care nurses during these transports is seemingly consistent.

Discharge from the ICU is facilitated once the critical care issues are resolved and the discharge criteria are met. The patient is then transferred to either a step-down unit, if institutionally available, or to the general ward, depending on its availability. The choice of room among those that are available is highly dependent on the financial capacity of the patient and family and their attending physician's preference. Although there are cases in which patients are discharged directly from the ICU, those are exemptions rather than the general trend.

Issues Within the Critical Care Unit

The complexities of cases present and the multidisciplinary approach used in the critical care unit generate unique issues within these units. Critical care nurses acting as patient advocates and providing most bedside care are at times witness to these issues. From the perspective of critical care nurses and within the context of the ICU and the Philippine health care system, the following are some of the prevalent issues within the critical care units.

Pain management

Pain is one of the most common signs seen and expected to be present in the ICU. It may arise from the patient's disease condition, present condition, or procedures done to the patient. Although the management of pain is one of the functions of critical care nurses, critical care nurses in the Philippines tend to use pharmacologic measures to alleviate pain, which is heavily reliant on the physician's management and orders. There seems to be an underutilization of nonpharmacologic measures and overreliance on drugs to control pain. This is further compounded by the practice of assessing only the severity of the pain, leaving behind the other aspects of the pain experience. Although there is a preference for pharmacologic pain management, there is a still a prevailing culture among Filipino health care providers of undermedicating patients who are experiencing pain. The inclination to use drugs found at the lower levels of the World Health Organization pain ladder and the underuse of opioids for pain management is still commonplace.[11,12] Although pain is a common occurrence in the ICU, little nursing research has been done to explore this phenomenon, its nature, management, and nursing implications, in the Philippines.

Management of delirium

Delirium is characterized by a disturbance in consciousness resulting in severe confusion and reduced awareness of surroundings.[13] It is often associated with poor health outcomes, neurocognitive impairment, prolonged length of stay in the ICU, prolonged mechanical ventilation, greater risks to safety related to self-extubation and falls, reduced health-related quality of life, as well as higher overall mortality rate.[14,15] Despite being a condition of growing concern in the ICU setting, especially for mechanically ventilated patients, little is still known about the prevalence of delirium among patients in ICUs in the Philippines. Although different tools for assessment are available for delirium, such as the Confusion Assessment Method for the ICU, its screening is still not part of routine care in the local ICU setting, thus delirium is frequently underdiagnosed.[16,17]

Provision of sleep

Disturbance of sleep in the ICU setting is influenced by illumination, noise (ie, alarms, monitors, staff voices), discomfort, anxiety, and various interventions done to the patient. The essentiality of sleep for the regeneration of the body is hampered, thus affecting the patient's recovery process and resulting in possible disorientation.[18] Although critical care nurses continuously monitor changes in the sleep pattern of patients in the ICU, there is no standard tool used in most of the units and most often these observations are merely endorsed to the incoming shift rather than properly documented in the patient's chart. Critical care nurses play an essential role in minimizing sleep disturbance by maximizing all activities to be done during daytime; bathing the patient before midnight; controlling room temperature, noise, and light; and positioning the patient based on their preference, which will promote a restful sleep. These activities are ideally done if the circumstances within the units permit, as some ICUs in government hospitals are not as spacious, well lit, and noise free as their private hospital counterparts. Administration of drugs solely to induce and fix the sleeping pattern is rarely done.

Patient rehabilitation

Within the setup among the ICUs in the Philippines, patients needing physical rehabilitation are formally referred to a rehabilitation team often led by a physician and composed mostly of physical and occupational therapists. Rehabilitation is often initiated as soon as the patient is stabilized and ready for therapy. Passive range-of-motion exercises are often done with the patient, whereas mobility and ambulation are rarely an occurrence within the ICU. These exercises are delegated to the physical rehabilitation team that visits the unit for each session. The critical care nurses seldom perform an active role during the therapy sessions except for preparing the patient by adjusting equipment and activities within the day and performing handover before and after the therapy session. During the active therapy session of their patient, critical care nurses will focus on their other patients, as they are assigned more than 1 patient most of the time. With the limitations of health care professionals conducting rehabilitation sessions and the emergence of Covid-19, telerehabilitation, a branch of telemedicine in which teleconference with the therapist on one side and the nurse tasked to assist the patient on the other, is slowly beginning to develop. Although this will increase the engagement of the nurse with patient's rehabilitation therapy, it will inevitably increase the nurse's workload as well. Institutions offering telerehabilitation are still limited in the country.[19,20]

Respiratory rehabilitation is always led by a physician, with nurses and the respiratory therapist acting as support personnel. Respiratory rehabilitation is achieved by various ventilatory weaning strategies based on protocols and physician's preference. Although other countries have established nurse-led ventilation-weaning protocols, with much success and good clinical outcomes,[21] its practice in the Philippines has yet to be observed or reported.

Quality and safety

With the promulgation of the Republic Act 7875 or the National Health Insurance Act of the Philippines, hospital institutions were mandated to establish quality assurance programs,[22] which has significantly led to the strict adherence to national standards as set by PhilHealth. International accreditations, such as the Joint Commission International, Canadian Hospital Accreditation, and Pathway to Excellence, were also sought by some hospitals on top of those given by Philhealth.[23] Most of these institutions are private hospitals. Although there are quality assurance and hospital-wide accreditations in place, there is none distinct for critical care units except if these units are part of "centers" especially built for specific diseases or medical conditions. Exemplars of these are the neurocritical care unit (NCCU) of Brain Specialty Centers designated by the Department of Health. These Brain Specialty Centers are projected to be on par with international standards, and will have a separate NCCU on top of their other ICUs.[24] Among these hospitals, few have started with their technological updates and have already acquired advance machine technologies, such as those used for targeted temperature management for improved neurologic outcomes.[25]

More recently, emphasis on health care provider safety from exposure to infection during handling and transport of patients has been raised. Health care providers are required to don appropriate personal protective equipment (PPE) as mandated by their hospital's infection control service. Departments in which the patient is to be transferred are alerted ahead of time of incoming patients to allow their staff ample time to don their own PPE. The shortest routes to these areas are used, and are usually cordoned off so that people, especially patients and visitors, are kept from crossing paths with suspected COVID-19 cases. It is also mentioned that portable diagnostic equipment, rather than patient transport to diagnostic areas, is given priority to minimize the exposure of others to possible infection.

Technology in Critical Care

Technology and its utilization in critical care varies from unit to unit and institution to institution. Advances in state-of-the-art technology still press an issue in the practice of most critical care nursing.[3] Advanced technologies, such as hemodynamic monitors, ventilators, and specialized equipment, such as extracorporeal membrane oxygenation, continuous electrocardiogram (cEEG), continuous renal replacement therapy, intracranial pressure (ICP) monitors, cooling and warming devices, perfusion machines, automated medicine cabinets, and nursing informatics are more widely available and used in private institutions as compared with government hospitals.

Inside the ICU units, each patient's headboard is equipped with inlets/outlets for oxygenation, and suctioning. Patients needing mechanical ventilation (MV) can be set up inside the room if rooms are available or beside the bed within their confined space. A small portable MV can be used as well during patient transport. Private ICUs have automated handheld ear thermometers and can be used with disposable ear probes. Since the pandemic, most hospitals acquired gun thermometers for their use.

Individual ICU beds are equipped with at least a bedside monitor for continuous vital signs, heart rhythm, and oxygen saturation tracking. Each monitor is connected to a central monitor that is visible in the nurse's station and most often monitored by the head nurse or a trained telemetry nurse if there is one in the institution,[6] whereas in other ICUs, the monitors are individualized per patient and there is no central monitoring system.[6] These monitors can be switched to a portable device when necessitating transport from one unit to another.

In light of the pandemic, a Filipino innovation for patient monitoring, called RxBox biomedical monitoring devices, was used in some government facilities handing patients with COVID-19. This portable device can provide monitoring comparable to other branded monitoring devices.[26]

Brain monitoring devices, such as ICP monitors and cEEGs, are now accessible in some ICUs, mostly from private institutions. ICP monitoring can be done invasively and noninvasively via a multidisciplinary facet. Invasive ICP monitoring with the application of monitoring devices can be applied if the device is available and warranted. Such devices can show numbers and ICP waves to monitor trends in pressures. Critical care nurses are part of the team that monitors these ICP readings, but nurses seem to be more reliant on the numerical values of the reading than the meaning of the waves and its trends, as some are not trained for this competency.

Several private institutions and a few government facilities are equipped with computerized medication management systems that are a part of their hospital information system (HIS). Most HISs also have integrated picture archiving and communications systems (PACS) in which members of the multidisciplinary team can view images of the diagnostic procedures, such as radiographs and scans. Some PACS vendors allow mobile access that is convenient for physicians to view their diagnostic images even if they are outside the hospital through a secured network.

Interprofessional Communication and Collaboration

The critical care team in most ICUs in the Philippines are primarily composed of physicians (intensivists, critical care specialists, residents) and nurses (bedside, charge, and head nurses). There is no advanced practice nurse in the Philippines, but all nurses working in the ICU are trained in basic critical care by either their respective institution or through other noninstitutional trainings. Other ICUs have respiratory therapists and clinical pharmacists as part of their team. Other health care professionals, such as rehabilitation therapists, dieticians, and medical technologists are called depending on the patient's needs and concerns. Social workers and chaplains are available for the whole hospital and are called depending on the request of the patient's family and the attending physicians. Social workers are often called to assist in locating additional funding for the patient, whereas chaplains are, most often than not, lay ministers from a Christian denomination either hired by the institution or serving on a voluntary basis. Although there are a significant number of non-Christian patients admitted in the ICU, provisions for referral for pastoral care from their religious denomination are lacking. With these, if the family wished for a non-Christian pastoral service, referrals need to be facilitated by them from outside the hospital. Individual ICUs have different guidelines on allowing persons not connected with the institution to perform chaplaincy within their unit; some allow it, whereas others prohibit it, citing safety, privacy, and infection control issues.

Given the complexity of care present in these units, interprofessional collaboration between various health care professionals is essential and has been found to significantly decrease mortality and morbidity rate among patients admitted in the ICU.[27] Critical care nurses in the Philippines play an instrumental role in maintaining the openness and collaborative atmosphere between and among various health care professionals caring for the patient. They provide significant input to other health care professionals managing the patient; their collective information provides a more holistic understanding of the patient's condition that is not viewed solely through each professional's disciplinary perspective. As nurses provide the longest bedside interaction and presence with the patient, they manage the schedules of other health care professionals so conflicts of schedules are prevented and all activities are bundled to provide more rest period for the patient. All referrals to other health care professionals will pass through the nurses and notification for referrals will be sent by them. Despite these vital roles that critical care nurses play within the ICU, their active participation during medical/interprofessional rounds or patient case analysis is still lacking. Most often, during these instances, the voices of the critical care nurses will be heard only when a question, commonly about a patient's vital signs, is directly asked of them.[28] Critical care nurses' communication with other health care providers outside the ICU team is limited to referral and endorsement with the patient's scheduled activities. In this sense, interprofessional communication seems to be present but active collaboration by the nurses needs further improvement.

Family involvement, end-of life choices, and palliative care
Most of the ICUs in the Philippines do not allow family members to stay with their patient but instead have a fixed visiting hour where they can check on their relatives. In most instances, family members stay in another private room, if they can afford it, or a room dedicated for all family members of all patients admitted in the ICU, or a spot in and/or around the hospital premises where announcements can be heard where they could be called in to provide decisions or personal provisions that the hospital cannot provide for. The first is common in private hospitals, whereas the last are almost exclusively found in government health institutions. This system seems to add to the overall burden and anxiety felt by the families of patients admitted in the ICU.[29,30]

During visitation hours, the critical care nurse assigned to the patient is often the health professional who gives updates to the patient's family. Most of the information conveyed within this interaction involves the patient's status, vital signs, and procedure done within the shift. Information deemed as "serious" by the nurse is not divulged to the family member but is referred to the available physician handling the patient so the information will be coming directly from the physician. This information may include the prognosis of the patient given the current situation, the current overall status of the patient, the professional advice for end-of-life decisions, and possibility of organ donation.[28–30]

The practice of organ donation varies among individual critical care units. Although there are laws and promulgations that facilitate its process, dilemmas usually occur when the living relative of the patient does not consent for harvesting of the organ to proceed.[31,32] In the absence of a last will or an advanced directive from the patient, the family would rather have the patient "intact and complete" than go through the process of organ donation.

Although there exists a presidential promulgation for the integration of palliative and hospital care in the Philippines, palliative care provisions are not functionally integrated in most local ICUs.[33] Most hospitals do not have a separate specialized team that specifically provides palliative care, and palliative care, as practiced in the ICU, is focused mostly on pain control and management. Provisions and referral for palliative care are not routinely coordinated or deliberately offered with the patient's family in the early stage of management, but they are usually informed by the time it involves end-of-life decisions.[29,30] For this reason, the Philippines is categorized as belonging to group 3a, those that have isolated provisions of palliative care.[34] This is one of the factors contributing to why the Philippines was considered as one of the worst countries to die in, ranking 78th of 80 countries in the 2015 Quality of Death study index.[35] This, along with insufficiency of public information, lack of training among health professionals, low interest in the field of palliative care, unwillingness of doctors to refer patients, absence of legal basis supporting palliative care, and scarcity of government stream for hospice funding, contribute to the current situation of palliative care in the Philippines, and is very much reflected in various local ICU units.[36]

Because of this prevailing system, end-of-life decisions within the critical care units are more heavily influenced by the physician's medical opinion rather than the result of the active participation of the patient's family members. This is compounded by the reality that most Filipinos do not have a living will or advance directive, owing to the prevailing belief that death is a taboo topic, thus the possibility of death is not openly discussed with their families.[37] End-of-life decisions are rarely discussed until such time when withdrawal of treatment is beginning to be considered.

The option for withdrawal of treatment is mostly decided by the patient's medical prognosis and the family's prevailing belief on the morality of withdrawing treatment. In the Philippines, where euthanasia is not legal and Christianity is a dominant religion, simple acts or measures, such as turning off the ventilator and giving opioids, could be perceived as tantamount to killing the patient. A common dilemma among family members who decided to withdraw treatment is who will turn off the patient's mechanical ventilator. These, among other misconceptions, serve as barriers in deciding to limit life-sustaining therapy in a dying patient.[29,30,38] Ultimately, the financial difficulties and burden brought about by high hospital bills will inevitably play a more significant role in deciding when to withdraw the treatment.

IMPLICATIONS AND FUTURE DIRECTIONS

A holistic approach is needed to continually uplift critical care nursing practice in the Philippines. Laws need to be created to promulgate the advancement of its practice and affect systemic change in the country's health care system that directly affects the processes inherent in various critical care units. Appropriate funding, prioritization for health, and directives on a national level are greatly needed. Albeit the practice of critical care nursing in the Philippines follows the international and regional standards, and the current lack of national competencies for critical care nurses may be one of the reasons for its delayed professional growth. Luckily, this lacking national standard is now being created through the collaborative efforts of critical care nurses, nursing leaders, and government instrumentalities.

Although critical care nurses in the Philippines are skilled in the technicalities of technologies in the ICU, and are competent in caring for the patient, there is a need to focus and improve their competencies on pain management, delirium recognition, interprofessional collaboration, and end-of-life decisions. Critical care nurses' training also should include communication skills, conflict resolution, and palliative care for them to become better empowered to fully fulfill their roles as a collaborative clinician and an active patient advocate.

DISCLOSURE

The authors have nothing to disclose.

REFERENCES

1. Porciuncula C, Blanco-Limpin ME, San Juan BG, et al, editors. Philippine Heart Center 30 years of heart care and compassion coffee table book. Quezon City: Philippine Heart Center; 2005.
2. Critical Care Nurses Association of the Philippines. Critical care nursing guidelines, standards and competencies. 2014. Available at: http://www.ccnapi.org/news-and-events/critical-care-nursing-guidelines-standards-and-competencies/. Accessed October 18, 2020.
3. Paguio JT, Banayat AC. Commentary on challenges to critical care nursing practice in the Philippines. sgrwfccn 2018;12(1):8–11.
4. Dayrit MM, Lagrada LP, Picazo OF, et al. The Philippines health system review. World Health Organization. India: Regional Office for South-East Asia; 2018. Available at: https://apps.who.int/iris/bitstream/handle/10665/274579/9789290226734-eng.pdf?sequence=1&isAllowed=y.
5. Picazo OF. Public hospital governance in the Philippines. In: Hort K, editors. Public Hospital Governance in Asia and the Pacific. Comparative Country Studies. World Health Organization; 2015:186-221. Available at: https://books.google.com.ph/books?id=WRiYjgEACAAJ.
6. Phua J, Faruq MO, Kulkarni AP, et al. Critical care bed capacity in Asian Countries and regions. Crit Care Med 2020;48(5):654–62.
7. UP COVID-19 Pandemic Response. Estimating local healthcare capacity to deal with COVID-19 case surge: analysis and recommendations. University of the Philippines Website; 2020. Available at: https://www.up.edu.ph/estimating-local-healthcare-capacity-to-deal-with-covid-19-case-surge-analysis-and-recommendations/. Accessed October 20, 2020.
8. Marshall JC, Bosco L, Adhikari NK, et al. What is an intensive care unit? A report of the task force of the World Federation of Societies of Intensive and Critical Care Medicine. J Crit Care 2017;37:270–6.
9. DOH-Philippines. Revised organizational structure and staffing standards for government hospitals. 2013. Available at: https://www.dbm.gov.ph/wp-content/uploads/Issuances/2013/Joint Circular 2013/DOH/Manual RSSGH_ 3 levels.pdf. Accessed October 1, 2020.
10. Samuelsson C, Thach Q. Nurses experiences on work-related health in the Philippines. 2018;(June):1-22. Available at: http://www.diva-portal.org/smash/get/diva2:1210360/FULLTEXT01.pdf. Accessed September 27, 2020.
11. Javier FO, Calimag MP. Opioid use in the Philippines - 20 years after the introduction of the WHO analgesic ladder. Eur J Pain Suppl 2007;1(1):19–22.
12. Galanti GA. Filipino attitudes toward pain medication. A lesson in cross-cultural care. West J Med 2000;173(4):278–9.
13. Cavallazzi R, Saad M, Marik PE. Delirium in the ICU: an overview. Ann Intensive Care 2012;2(1):1–11.
14. Gulay C, Saranza G, Tuble G, et al. Neurocognitive outcome of patients with delirium in the intensive care units at a tertiary government hospital. Philipp J Chest Dis 2017;18(2):14–21.
15. Ofquila RM, Ybanez A, Llamedo M, et al. Health-related quality of life and cognitive functioning of intensive care unit (ICU) survivors with delirium and non-delirium states from a Philippine Provincial Hospital. Int J Health Sci Res 2016;6(6):301–6. Available at: https://www.ijhsr.org/IJHSR_Vol.6_Issue.6_June2016/49.pdf.

16. Tuble GC, Saranza GM, Albay AB, et al. Prevalence of delirium in patients admitted at intensive care units of Philippine General Hospital. Philipp J Chest Dis 2015;16(3):27–33.

17. Tanuatmadja AP, Vea JR. Prevalence of delirium and its clinical outcome in adult Filipino patients admitted in the intensive care unit. J Med Health 2019;2(4):920–9.

18. Miranda-Ackerman RC, Lira-Trujillo M, Gollaz-Cervantez AC, et al. Associations between stressors and difficulty sleeping in critically ill patients admitted to the intensive care unit: a cohort study. BMC Health Serv Res 2020;20(1). https://doi.org/10.1186/s12913-020-05497-8.

19. Leochico CFD, Espiritu AI, Ignacio SD, et al. Challenges to the emergence of tele-rehabilitation in a developing country: a systematic review. Front Neurol 2020;11. https://doi.org/10.3389/fneur.2020.01007.

20. Carl CF. Adoption of telerehabilitation in a developing country before and during the COVID-19 pandemic. Ann Phys Rehabil Med 2020;11. https://doi.org/10.1016/j.rehab.2020.06.001.

21. Hirzallah FM, Alkaissi A, do Céu Barbieri-Figueiredo M. A systematic review of nurse-led weaning protocol for mechanically ventilated adult patients. Nurs Crit Care 2019;24(2):89–96.

22. Maramba J. Conference report first national meeting on quality assurance in healthcare in the Philippines. Int J Qual Health Care 1997;9(5):381–2.

23. Asinas-Tan M, Leonardo J, Aldana E, et al. Implementation of quality improvement strategies for better patient care. Int J Integr Care 2016;16(6):20.

24. Health Systems Development and Management Support Division, Health Facility Development Bureau. Stakeholder's consultation: expanding access to brain specialty care. 2019. Available at: http://caro.doh.gov.ph/wp-content/uploads/2019/11/Brain-Centers-lecture-materials.pdf. Accessed September 26, 2020.

25. HealthSolutions installs first-ever BARD Arctic Sun at QMMC. The Manila Times. Available at: https://www.manilatimes.net/2019/03/20/public-square/healthsolutions-installs-first-ever-bard-arctic-sun-at-qmmc/528088/. 2019.

26. Sambatyon E. UP and DOST-developed RxBox vital signs monitor for COVID-19 patients now in use at Philippine General Hospital. Good News Pilipinas. Available at: https://www.goodnewspilipinas.com/up-and-dost-developed-rxbox-vital-signs-monitor-for-covid-19-patients-now-in-use-at-philippine-general-hospital/. 2020. Accessed September 27, 2020.

27. Curtis JR, Cook DJ, Wall RJ, et al. Intensive care unit quality improvement: a "how-to" guide for the interdisciplinary team. Crit Care Med 2006;34(1):211–8.

28. Martinez RCKP. "Of technical competence, perceived autonomy and relational expertise": Understanding professional identity among nurses working in a stroke unit. 2019. https://doi.org/10.31235/osf.io/dh65f.

29. Berdeguel RE, Martinez RCKP. "Hope Within Hopelessness": The lives of families whose member is on {DNR} (Do Not Resuscitate) Status. 2019. https://doi.org/10.31235/osf.io/geusd.

30. Sumaguingsing R, Martinez RCKP. "Swinging Pendulum": Lives of Family Members Caring for A Dying Relative. 2019. https://doi.org/10.31235/osf.io/tqzp6.

31. Organ donation act of 1991. Congress of the Philippines. 1992. Available at: https://www.officialgazette.gov.ph/1992/01/07/republic-act-no-7170/. Accessed October 1, 2020.

32. Department of Health. National policy on palliative and hospice care in the Philippines. Philippines. 2015. Available at: https://www.doh.gov.ph/sites/default/files/health_programs/AO2015-0052. Accessed September 26, 2020.

33. World Health Organization. Global atlas of palliative care at the end of life. World-wide Palliative Care Alliance 2014. Available at: https://www.who.int/nmh/Global_Atlas_of_Palliative_Care.pdf. Accessed September 26, 2020.
34. Worldwide Palliative Care Alliance, World Health Organization. Global atlas of palliative care at the end of life. Worldwide Palliative Care Alliance; 2014. Available at: https://www.who.int/nmh/Global_Atlas_of_Palliative_Care.pdf.
35. The 2015 quality of death index. 2015. Available at: https://eiuperspectives. economist.com/sites/default/files/images/2015 Quality of Death Index Country Profiles_Oct 6 FINAL.pdf. Accessed October 2, 2020.
36. Department of Health. Palliative and hospice report Philippines. 2008. Available at: https://www.doh.gov.ph/sites/default/files/health_programs/Palliative and Hospice Report Philippines.pdf. Accessed October 2, 2020.
37. Soriano GP, Calong KAC. Religiosity, spirituality, and death anxiety among Filipino older adults: a correlational study. J Death Dying 2020. https://doi.org/10. 1177/0030222820947315. 003022282094731.
38. Manalo MFC. End-of-life decisions about withholding or withdrawing therapy: medical, ethical, and religio-cultural considerations. Palliat Care Res Treat 2013;7:1–5. PCRT.S10796.

The Glasgow Coma Scale
A European and Global Perspective on Enhancing Practice

Neal F. Cook, PhD, MSc, PG Dip Nurse Education, PG Cert, Dip Aromatherapy, RN,
Lecturer/Practice Educator, Specialist Practitioner Adult, PFHEA

KEYWORDS

- Glasgow Coma Scale education • Neuroscience nurses • Person-centered care

KEY POINTS

- Although the Glasgow Coma Scale is a well-established and effective tool in clinical practice, there remains inconsistency in its use, largely because of variances in educational approach and the lack of internationally accepted, unambiguous practice standards.
- Human factors have traditionally not been addressed in education on the Glasgow Coma Scale or in related practice guidelines, despite such factors having a direct impact on practitioners, patients, and their relatives.
- An opportunity exists, and needs to be taken, to develop explicit, unambiguous, interprofessional, international standards for use of the Glasgow Coma Scale, underpinned by evidence.
- The implementation of such interprofessional, international standards should be framed within an agreed on educational framework.
- The success of both the educational framework and the international standards should be evaluated through further research.

INTRODUCTION

Since its inception in 1974 as a 14-point scale, and subsequent modification into a 15-point scale, the Glasgow Coma Scale (GCS)[1] has stood the test of time as the most commonly used tool to assess level of consciousness globally.[2] Indeed, in 2014, it was relaunched with modification to the wording and guidance for its use; how universally adopted the relaunched version has been is yet to be seen some 6 years later. What is clear, is that the GCS, through time, has seen variation, undergone scrutiny through a plethora of studies, and although commonly adopted and accepted, continues to have an air of ambiguity around its use as a result of a perceived lack of clarity

School of Nursing, Ulster University, Londonderry BT48 7JL, Northern Ireland
E-mail address: nf.cook@ulster.ac.uk
Twitter: @NealFCook (N.F.C.)

Crit Care Nurs Clin N Am 33 (2021) 89–99
https://doi.org/10.1016/j.cnc.2020.10.005
0899-5885/21/Crown Copyright © 2020 Published by Elsevier Inc. All rights reserved.
ccnursing.theclinics.com

in certain aspects of its use. A key question is whether the tool itself is at the heart of any issues around its use, or the guidelines, standards, and education that surround its use.

THE GLASGOW COMA SCALE OVER TIME

Although the GCS has endured over time, it has not done so without criticism and some controversy, for example, on how to elicit a response to pain, or indeed pressure as it is now referred to in the 2014 relaunched version. The change from response to pain to pressure alone leaves us with a question about whether we are indeed assessing a response to pressure or pain, or indeed the rationale for the change itself. Criticism has also been reflected in its perceived complexity, its inability to discriminate sufficiently at midrange score level, and its potential inaccuracy to reflect arousability and awareness when a person is intubated or nonverbal[3,4]; a person may be entirely aware and fully arousable when intubated, but the tool does not account for this. Although there has been criticism in relation to interrater reliability, a systematic review of 53 studies in 2016 concluded that 85% of findings in research studies, considered rigorous, demonstrated *substantial* reliability; 77% showed high reproducibility[5] (kappa statistic >0.6). Considering tools are used in practice to support assessment and inform, not replace, clinical judgment, the result of this analysis is impressive.

In reviewing the evidence base for use of the GCS over time, Braine and Cook[4] concluded that the tool has been adopted interprofessionally, facilitating effective communication and understanding of a person's level of consciousness because of the use of a common, understood clinical language and measurement. Indeed, a variety of other tools for assessing consciousness have been developed over time, many having clinical credibility, but none have been as universally adopted and sustained over time as the GCS, despite many, often varied, criticisms around interrater reliability. One example is the Full Outline of Unresponsiveness score, which, in 1 study, showed a better predictive power for mortality,[6] but has not been universally adopted. Braine and Cook[4] clearly identify that issues around interrater reliability are multifactorial; the level of skill to use the tool and clarity about how to use the tool clearly impact on interrater reliability, factors that are indeed separate to issues around the construct and nature of the tool itself. As with any skill in assessment, skills enhance over time and with experience; the challenge here is consistency in the education, policy, and guidelines as to how to use the tool. Otherwise, there is a risk of miseducating people to develop expertise in how to do something incorrectly. As both Braine and Cook[5] and Cook and colleagues[7] highlight, there currently exists no universally adopted and accepted standard for education on the GCS and its safe and effective use; this is clearly a problem. The results of the study by Cook and colleagues[7] clearly show that despite experience, education, and familiarity with the tool over time, practices varied, and there was a clear message from respondents (n = 273) in the study that nurses wanted clearer, universal guidelines. Furthermore, respondents also wanted the tool to be considered within the context of professional, person-centered practice. For example, the respondents clearly expressed concern and anxiety over the family's experience of seeing painful stimuli applied and were conflicted about the application of painful stimuli when they perceived it as distressing for the person. No publication or education material to date was identified that dealt with these concerns. In addition, the plethora of existing publications in the past 40 years has led to nuances and traditions around the use of the GCS, often containing guidelines unsupported by evidence.[4] Of concern is that there is evidence that illustrates that this confusion can cause potential harm at an international level[7]; Cook and colleagues[7] found that practices varied internationally, and within countries, and that participants were not clear about how to apply a painful stimulus. Great variation in practices was found and, indeed, some inappropriate and ineffective methods of applying painful stimuli that could lead to harm; complications were found in the use of supraorbital pressure, sternal rub, and nail bed pressure, among others. This study was the first known to be published that documented such complications and further highlights the need for consistency.

STANDARDIZATION OF THE GLASGOW COMA SCALE

It would be reasonable to question, at this stage, why the GCS should be set out as an area where standardization is necessary. In 2016 (most recent European Union [EU] statistics at the time of writing), 3.2% of all deaths in the 28 countries of the EU were related to accidents, more than 163,000 deaths[8] (updated November 2019). These accidents typically would have a neurologic element (motor vehicle accidents, falls, drowning, poisoning, and so forth). Further exploration at the European level makes it clear that traumatic brain injury (TBI) accounts for almost 1.4 million hospital admissions.[9] This amount represents almost 1.4 million people requiring reliable assessment of level of consciousness in order to prevent, where possible, associated potential deaths by being able to respond rapidly to any deterioration (12 per 100,000 adjusted mortality[9] and 3.3–28.10 per 100,000 population per year[10]). Furthermore, those who survive their TBI must be considered. It is known that neurologic disorders are the leading group of disability-adjusted life-years (DALYs) (2015 data[11]), with a 7.4% increase in DALYs in a 25-year period. The trends in the data support that neurologic disorders are not becoming less prevalent, despite advances in care and interventions; the need for expert knowledge, education, and clarity in using core tools in practice is therefore amplified going forward. In addition, the nervous system is one of two primary control and regulation systems in the body, the endocrine system being the other, and the two are highly integrated. It is therefore vitally important that nurses can undertake assessment of the nervous system, with level of consciousness being fundamental to assessing and monitoring any deterioration in neurologic functioning/status. Alongside that, consistency and standardization are essential to the translation of assessment across settings and professionals.

GLASGOW COMA SCALE AS PART OF PREREGISTRATION NURSING CURRICULA

The practice of each nurse is shaped by their education and the culture of practice within which they learn. If you are taught something incorrectly, and this is reinforced in practice by seeing similar practices, then we can expect to see this practice continued, taught to others, and be underpinned by a belief that this practice is correct. Evidence shows us that newly qualified nurses will reshape their beliefs and professional identities under organizational pressures and through role-modeling of practices from their experienced peers[12]; nurses often adapt to the culture of practice they work in, which necessitates that we role-model best practice. In addition, when the use of a tool spans disciplines, as can be seen with the GCS (eg, nurses, paramedics, and medical staff use it frequently), then the need for explicit clarity and consistency in approach is paramount for the translation to practice and interpretation of findings to be accurate. Preregistration education is the most effective place to start such education so as to shape the knowledge and skills of the novice practitioner in order that they recognize best practice and can make sufficient critical analysis of what is role-modeled in practice.

The inconsistency in the use and education of the GCS is not a new observation, although evidence has lacked some explicit detail to that uncovered by Cook and colleagues[7]; this study was a snapshot that merits further research to expand to larger numbers to gain a more in-depth analysis of the global picture. Iacono and colleagues[13] also identified inconsistency in neurologic assessment as an issue in their hospital, setting out a program of education to standardize assessment across all nurses; it is not clear why a multidisciplinary approach was not taken in their intervention to address this if the interprofessional translation of the use of tools in neurologic assessment is to be consistent. Although not formally evaluated in a measurable way, feedback from participants (of whom the total is not reported) indicated increased confidence and knowledge. The translation to practice, however, was not explored, and it is this translation that is essential; such assessment of practice could be argued as more likely to occur if embedded in preregistration education. Verbalizing confidence is not the same as correctly undertaking, albeit a very important factor in competence. However, in effect, this form of standardization, although it appears effective, came after these nurses completed their preregistration education. If preregistration education is preparing students to be effective registrants, it could be argued that such education is failing these students in providing education and skills development in the use of the most universally accepted clinical assessment tool in neurologic assessment.

Similarly, Enriquez and colleagues[14] used an educational approach to standardize practice (n = 20), demonstrating their educational intervention improved application of the GCS and increased confidence. Although they refer to generating standards in their publication, they effectively standardized the education, which may achieve consistency in that area, but not necessarily achieve standardization of correct practices, particularly in the absence of any definitive publication of agreed standards in this regard. Practice can be consistently incorrect as much as it can be consistently correct. A further UK study in 2019 with medical and nursing professionals yielded that only 9.7% of participants correctly used the GCS (n = 55)[15]; following an educational intervention, this increased to 71%, showing the power of education to transform practice, but not within preregistration education. However, Dubey and Kumar[16] demonstrated that a computer-assisted teaching program significantly increased knowledge on the GCS in final-year preregistration nursing students (n = 60), highlighting that early educational intervention can be successful at this stage of education. Educational endeavors clearly have the potential to maximize consistency; the missing piece is an international standard to ensure what we are teaching is accurate and consistent to quality assure such education. Fundamentally, it is also evident that there is a desire to standardize and perfect practice, as seen in the studies cited; the development of such standards therefore has great potential to feed into practices that desire consistency and best practice. However, matters cannot stop at standardized practice. It can also be concluded from these studies that, in some cases, intervention is coming after these professionals have completed their preregistration education, a case of an undoing of incorrect practices and relearning correct practices. Applying standards through an effective educational approach at the right time in the development of health care professionals is essential, and the evidence indicates this should occur at preregistration level.

In considering the education delivered around the GCS, a consistent approach also must consider the expectation set for preregistration nursing education. The need for a consistent approach to nurse education is ever more important within an increasingly global nursing workforce as a result of international mobility of nurses and a variety of schemes in countries that facilitate the assimilation of internationally educated nurses into their workforce.[17] In Europe, there is a degree of standardization in those countries that are a member state of the EU under the EU directive 2005/36/EC.[18] In essence, this directive recognizes equivalency of education for nurses educated on programs that are confirmed against this directive. However, a quick analysis of how well this standardizes matters can be clearly illustrated when we examine education around the GCS in Europe alone. Although the EU directive does not provide explicit detail in relation to neurologic assessment, national standards could provide this, although this approach would still require the existence of a universally accepted standard for education and use of the GCS. In the United Kingdom, the Nursing and Midwifery Council have specified in their 2018 standards for preregistration education[19(p33)] that nurses must be able to undertake a whole body systems assessment, including neurologic status, and *undertaking, responding to, and interpreting neurologic observations and assessments*. Meeting such a standard would necessitate use of the GCS, given its location within such assessment. In the Republic of Ireland, national standards are less prescriptive, with education standards specifying the need to be able to care for the unconscious person[20]; assessing level of consciousness would therefore be implicit. Neurologic assessment is not set out in standards for preregistration education in many countries of Europe, for example, Spain, Poland, Belgium, North Macedonia. Despite an EU directive for nursing education and a recognition of qualification, at the granular level, consistency and equivalency are not present in specific aspects of practice. An educational framework for consistency around GCS is therefore essential to achieve consistency.

In the Republic of Ireland, a National Clinical Programme for Neurology exists with the intention of being a framework for practice that follows international best practice, delivered within an integrated service approach.[21] This framework recognizes that neurosciences is a distinct, specialist area of practice whereby it is essential to underpin practice with evidence-informed practices and education. Although the program refers to developing advanced nurse practitioners, there is recognition of the absence of a national education framework for neurosciences, including for nurses. It therefore must be questioned how an integrated approach to service could be achieved without clear standardization of education in the related health professions. Indeed, if the findings of Cook and colleagues[7] are to be taken cognizance of, the use of the GCS in itself illustrates the lack of unified approach to education for its effective use, and that is for neuroscience nurses alone. Models of care need to be underpinned with effective education to be effective, and we must begin with what we teach our future workforce from the outset. If practice is confused, varied, and potentially harmful, as elicited by Cook and colleagues,[7] then what is role-modeled and reinforced to students must be considered, as it may perpetuate the situation. Indeed, the EU directive for preregistration nurse education (European Directive 2005/36/EC)[18] does not provide explicit requirements around specific aspects of practice, but more high-level requirements that still leave room for great variance. Utilising a high-level standards approach, within explicit detailed expectations, leaves it up to EU member countries to create their own level of standard to create a degree of consistency, or indeed for the foci of education to be set at curricula level. Although being prescriptive can be confining and restrictive for courses at the level of higher education, the lack of standardization in education certainly contributes to the variances seen in the practices of the use of the GCS.

In 2018, Vink and colleagues,[22] in a pan Europe study (n = 331), identified that assessment of consciousness was a daily activity for 95% of bedside neuroscience nurses with an estimated median frequency of 6 times per shift, and the GCS being the most commonly used tool. Most respondents (84.9%) had training/education in use of the GCS, but these were diverse, echoed in the findings of Cook and colleagues[7]; both studies support the need for standardization of education and use.

Of note is that 15.1% of neuroscience nurses had no training or education in the use of the GCS, despite its frequent use.[22] This finding is within the context of the 2019 study by Cook and colleagues[7] illustrating 31% of neuroscience nurses had no neuroscience education at all; an earlier study by Braine and Cook[23] identified 7% of neuroscience nurses as having no neuroscience-specific education. This finding creates a picture of reducing education in a climate of increasing incidence of neurologic disorders and only further supports that training programs and standards/guidelines need to be universally consistent and explicit if the variances in practice identified by both Vink and colleagues[22] and Cook and colleagues[7] are to be addressed. Globally, this picture is of similar concern, with only 5.2% of nurses (n = 115) in a study undertaken in Ghana demonstrating good knowledge on application of the GCS using scenarios.[24] A study in India found similar poor knowledge, with 33.1% of respondents (n = 154) having a good level of knowledge of the GCS.[25] A Saudi Arabian study in 2019 also identified inconsistencies in practice in using the GCS, but not the frequency of these.[26] Indeed, the article provides an algorithm that perpetuates variations from those normally undertaken in practice, such as asking the person their name and the current time; knowledge of name is not an accurate representation of awareness and knowledge of the current time is difficult for most people to get right. Guidance on determining confusion or inappropriate words is ambiguous and not consistent with the criteria for these elements, and the article perpetuates the confusion that exists between the use of a peripheral or central painful stimulus as identified by Braine and Cook.[4] Confusingly, Catangui[26] also included pupillary assessment as part of GCS assessment, when it is not a component of the scale. A 2019 study in Saudi Arabia showed that 69% of 149 nurses had no education on the use of the GCS.[27] The investigators state that results from their study contradict those of other studies in that there was no statistically significant association between educational attainment and knowledge of the GCS. However, the research was conducted using a questionnaire, which is provided in the publication, but of which the validity is not determined. The relationship between the questionnaire and the ability to accurately use the GCS is not established, and it is highly questionable as to whether the data from the questionnaire could represent such a correlation. In this respect, how useful the results are is questionable. What remains clear, however, is that the inconsistencies and continued dissemination of variances in practice remain an issue globally.

PERSON-CENTEREDNESS AND THE GLASGOW COMA SCALE

In considering any approach to education and practice, we need to consider the values held by the profession to ensure what we teach is contextual and aligned with those values. Nursing has long held caring and compassion at its core, and so the concerns raised by nurses in the study by Cook and colleagues[7] about causing distress to apply a painful stimulus and the secondary distress this may cause family are unsurprising, albeit that they have not been previously voiced in other studies on the GCS. Although unsurprising, they create a challenge for education and practice that cannot be ignored. How we prepare nurses to be able to deal with this distress and concern have not, it would seem, been considered a core component of GCS education to date. Emotionally challenging aspects of practice must be underpinned with rationale, discussion, and resolution as to how to manage these. In the United Kingdom, the Nursing and Midwifery Council[19(p9)] (the UK regulatory body for nursing) requires that, for a nurse to be proficient, they must be emotionally intelligent and resilient. In doing so, they must be *"capable of explaining the rationale that influences their judgments and decisions in routine, complex and challenging situations."* In teaching to apply a painful stimulus, we therefore need to do so within the context of a person-centered profession, facilitating nurses to deal with the complexity of emotions that may arise with this challenging aspect of their practice.

The culture of nursing has increasingly embraced the concept of person-centeredness, whereby we move beyond procedures and protocols and consider the people involved across the spectrum; how we work with each other, how we consider the world of the person in our care and the wider extension of that care in terms of their family, and indeed, the communities that people live in. Indeed, person-centeredness is increasingly an international priority, evident within the World Health Organization's strategy for People Centered and Integrated Health Services.[28,29] In considering the person-centered elements of this aspect of practice, we cannot ignore the issues around moral distress that may arise. In considering moral distress in this context, such distress may arise in circumstances whereby the nurse knows they need to apply a painful stimulus to determine the neurologic response, but is conscious of the perception of another (eg, a relative) as to the appropriateness of causing distress through pain for the purposes of assessment. The perception of the other may be a factor in preventing them from applying the painful stimulus. Equally, there may be unexplored cultural factors in what is an increasingly diverse workforce and whether cultural values permit applying pain as being justifiable in any circumstance. Pendry[30] recognizes that internal constraints originating from nurses' belief systems have not traditionally been captured in definitions of moral distress and yet the conflict of applying a painful stimulus clearly presented concerns for nurses in the study by Cook and colleagues.'[7] When a personal belief system signals to that person that it is wrong to inflict pain and distress, but the undertaking of an accurate neurologic assessment may require it, the conditions for moral distress are created.[31] Dealing with moral distress on an interprofessional level has been found to be beneficial to combat it, protecting health care professionals from burnout and detachment and from leaving their profession.[31] The knowledge that interventions around moral distress can effectively support nurses, and it is ethically right to do so, advocates the necessity to address this matter, not just for nurses, but also in consideration of all health care professionals whose practice involves using the GCS.

THE WAY FORWARD

It is clear from the evidence and discussions presented in this article that an effective strategy is needed to tackle issues around consistent and safe use of the GCS; it is a well-established tool that has proven itself, over time, to be important in assessment and monitoring of neurologic status. However, there is a clear need for standardization in the use of the tool through education approaches that are standardized and practice guidelines that are clear and explicit and that cite the evidence base. Furthermore, the human factors that impact use must be acknowledged and addressed within these in order to recognize, validate, and support practitioners in the use of techniques that potentially cause them, their patients, and relatives, distress.

The starting point for this must first be through consensus in creating a set of widely agreed on standards around the use of the GCS. For example, what are the acceptable methods of pain application and why? The greater the collaboration and agreement, the more effective they can be in standardizing practice and preventing harm through inconsistent use of the tool and unsafe use of techniques (ie, in applying painful stimuli). Authentic, collaborative co-design also creates the potential to formulate a consensus approach to dealing with those factors that are distressing. There exists the opportunity to achieve this through national and international organizations for nursing (eg, the World Federation of Neuroscience Nurses, the European Association of Neuroscience Nurses, the Australasian Neuroscience Nurses Association) and potentially in collaboration with medical colleagues in similar organizations (eg, World Federation of Neurosurgical Societies). The second proposed stage is then to agree on the most effective educational approach, including recommendations on whether such education should lie within preregistration education or at a postregistration/ postqualifying level. A collective view of the evidence suggests that this should be at preregistration level in the first instance. The third factor to be considered is the ongoing research necessary to determine whether such an approach has been effective in enhancing practice and in dealing with the ambiguity faced by practitioners (**Fig. 1**). Similar approaches have been effective in other practice specialties, one being standards developed by The International Continence Society for precision around practices in lower-urinary-tract dysfunction, removing ambiguity by being explicit and logical, but also by dealing with the human factors involved.[32]

In creating international standards for GCS use and education, which will be monitored and adapted based on sound evidence, there is a commitment given to enhancing the quality of care through the following[33]:

- Raising political awareness of the relevance of standards and quality
- Creating a vision of enhanced care by coming together globally to shape practice
- Creating and implementing standards that seek to enhance care quality
- Measuring the impact of processes to determine their effectiveness and enhance the evidence base to inform the further enhancement of practice and through creating a culture of enquiry.

Palm and colleagues[33] advocate this approach is aligned to creating the conditions for equitable access to health care of appropriate quality by the Convention on Human Rights and Biomedicine[34] and to create a culture of universality, equity, and solidarity.[35]

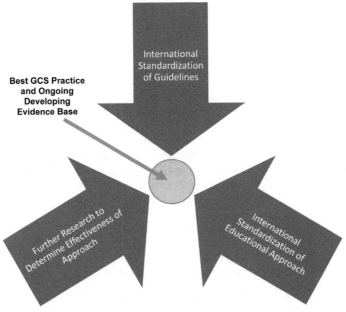

Fig. 1. Enhancing GCS practices: the way forward.

SUMMARY

Achieving best practice is a continual journey, one that is smoother and more direct when there is a roadmap set out. Although the GCS has made such a positive contribution to the care of people with neurologic orders, there has been an absence of a clear roadmap for its use. Various attempts have been made over the years to be clearer about the use of the tool, but with the GCS in its fifth decade of use, there remains issues around inconsistency that originate from a lack of a unified, consistent approach to education and practice. In an age of global health care practices and networking, an opportunity exists to create a standardized approach to the use of the GCS and the underpinning educational approach. Fundamentally, this would enable such an approach to be cognizant and responsive to the human factors involved, framing practice within a person-centered context.

CLINICS CARE POINTS

- Accuracy of use of the GCS is varied and inconsistent and requires a robust approach by educators and health care professionals alike.
- Human factors have traditionally been absent from education around use of the GCS; the impact of using the tool on the person, their loved ones, and the nurse must be considered and addressed in both education and practice.

DISCLOSURE

The author has nothing to disclose.

REFERENCES

1. Teasdale G, Jennett B. Assessment of coma and impaired consciousness: a practical scale. Lancet 1974;304(7872):81–4.
2. Teasdale G, Maas A, Lecky F, et al. The Glasgow Coma Scale at 40 years: standing the test of time. Lancet Neurol 2014;13(8):844–54.
3. Haukoos JS, Gill MR, Rabon RE, et al. Validation of the Simplified Motor Score for the prediction of brain injury outcomes after trauma. Ann Emerg Med 2007;50(1): 18–24.
4. Braine ME, Cook N. The Glasgow Coma Scale and evidence-informed practice: a critical review of where we are and where we need to be. J Clin Nurs 2017; 26(1–2):280–93.
5. Reith FC, Van den Brande R, Synnot A, et al. The reliability of the Glasgow Coma Scale: a systematic review. Intensive Care Med 2016;42(1):3–15.
6. Jalali R, Rezaei M. A comparison of the Glasgow Coma Scale score with full outline of unresponsiveness scale to predict patients' traumatic brain injury outcomes in intensive care units. Crit Care Res Pract 2014. https://doi.org/10. 1155/2014/289803. Article ID 289803.
7. Cook NF, Braine ME, Trout R. Nurses' understanding and experience of applying painful stimuli when assessing components of the Glasgow Coma Scale. J Clin Nurs 2019;28(21–22):3827–39.

8. Eurostat. Causes and occurrence of deaths in the EU. Luxembourg (Europe): Eurostat; 2019. Available at: https://ec.europa.eu/eurostat/web/products-eurostat-news/-/DDN-20190716-1. Accessed May 14, 2020.

9. Majdan M, Plancikova D, Brazinova A, et al. Epidemiology of traumatic brain injuries in Europe: a cross-sectional analysis. Lancet Public Health 2016;1(2): e76–83.

10. Brazinova A, Rehorcikova V, Taylor MS, et al. Epidemiology of traumatic brain injury in Europe: a living systematic review. J Neurotrauma 2016;33:1–30.

11. Feigin VL, Abajobir AA, Abate KH, et al. Global, regional, and national burden of neurological disorders during 1990–2015: a systematic analysis for the Global Burden of Disease Study 2015. Lancet Neurol 2017;16(11):877–97.

12. Hunter K, Cook C. Role-modelling and the hidden curriculum: new graduate nurses' professional socialisation. J Clin Nurs 2018;27(15–16):3157–70.

13. Iacono LA, Wells C, Mann-Finnerty K. Standardizing neurological assessments. J Neurosci Nurs 2014;46(2):125–32.

14. Enriquez CM, Chisholm KH, Madden LK, et al. Glasgow Coma Scale: generating clinical standards. J Neurosci Nurs 2019;51(3):142–6.

15. Jeffery J, Mussa M, Stirling E, et al. The Glasgow Coma Scale: do we know how to assess? J Orthop Surg 2019;2(1):65–8.

16. Dubey N, Kumar N. Assess the effectiveness of computer assisted teaching (CAT) on knowledge gain about GCS with coma patient among B. Sc. Nursing 3rd year students of selected nursing colleges at Bhopal, Madhya Pradesh, India. Trends in Nursing Administration and Education 2019;8(1):1–6.

17. Sherwood GD, Shaffer FA. The role of internationally educated nurses in a quality, safe workforce. Nurs Outlook 2014;62(1):46–52.

18. European Parliament. Directive 2005/36/EC of the European Parliament and of the Council of 7 September 2005 on the recognition of professional qualifications. Official Journal of the European Union 2005;255:22–142. Available at: https://eur-lex.europa.eu/LexUriServ/LexUriServ.do?uri=OJ:L:2005:255:0022:0142:EN:PDF. Accessed May 5, 2020.

19. Nursing and Midwifery Council (NMC). Future nurse: Standards of proficiency for registered nurses. London: NMC; 2018.

20. Nursing and Midwifery Board of Ireland. Nurse registration programmes standards and requirements. Dublin (Ireland): NMBI; 2016.

21. Health Service Executive (HSE). National clinical programme for neurology – model of care. Dublin (Ireland): HSE; 2016.

22. Vink P, Tulek Z, Gillis K, et al. Consciousness assessment: a questionnaire of current neuroscience nursing practice in Europe. J Clin Nurs 2018;27(21–22): 3913–9.

23. Braine ME, Cook N. An evaluation of post-registration neuroscience focused education and neuroscience nurses' perceived educational needs. Nurse Educ Today 2015;35(11):1069–74.

24. Alhassan A, Fuseini AG, Musah A. Knowledge of the Glasgow Coma Scale among nurses in a tertiary hospital in Ghana. Nurs Res Pract 2019;2019:1–7.

25. Sedain P, Bhusal MK. Knowledge regarding Glasgow Coma Scale (GCS) among nurses. Journal of College of Medical Sciences-Nepal 2019;15(4):276–81.

26. Catangui E. Improving Glasgow Coma Scale (GCS) competency of nurses in one acute stroke unit-a Nursing Initiative Project. J Nurs Pract 2019;3(1):109–15.

27. Albougami A. Exploring nurses' knowledge of the Glasgow Coma Scale in intensive care and emergency departments at a tertiary hospital in Riyadh City, Saudi Arabia. Malaysian J Nurs 2019;11(2):23–30.

28. World Health Organization. WHO global strategy on people-centred and integrated health services. Geneva (Swizerland): WHO; 2015.
29. Ward A, Eng C, McCue V, et al. What matters versus what's the matter–exploring perceptions of person-centred practice in nursing and physiotherapy social media communities: a qualitative study. International Practice Development Journal 2018;8(2). https://doi.org/10.19043/ipdj.82.003. article 3.
30. Pendry PS. Moral distress: recognizing it to retain nurses. Nurs Econ 2007; 25(4):217.
31. Browning ED, Cruz JS. Reflective debriefing: a social work intervention addressing moral distress among ICU nurses. Journal of Social Work in End-of-life & Palliative Care 2018;14(1):44–72.
32. Drake MJ, Abrams P. A commentary on expectations of healthcare professionals when applying the international continence society standards to basic assessment of lower urinary tract function. Neurourol Urodyn 2018;37(S6):S7–12.
33. Palm W, Peeters M, Garel P, et al. International and EU governance and guidance for national healthcare quality strategies. In: Busse R, Klazinga N, Panteli D, et al, editors. Improving healthcare quality in Europe. London: World Health Organization; 2019. p. 63–102.
34. Dommel FW, Alexander D. The convention on human rights and biomedicine of the Council of Europe. Kennedy Inst Ethics J 1997;7(3):259–76.
35. Council of the European Union. Council conclusions on common values and principles in European Union health systems. Official Journal of the European Union 2006;146:1–3.

Care of the Patient with Acquired Brain Injury in Latin America and the Caribbean

Stefany Ortega-Perez, RN, MSc, PhD[a],*,
María Consuelo Amaya-Rey, RN, BS, FNP, MSN, PhD[b],
Virginia Soto Lesmes, RN, MSN, PhD[b]

KEYWORDS

- Latin America • Traumatic brain injury • Stroke • Three delays model
- Neuroscience nursing • Nursing care

KEY POINTS

- In Latin American and Caribbean (LAC) region, specific characteristics such as models of health care systems and risk factors may influence the patient's outcome.
- Important delays exist in seeking care, reaching care, and receiving care and are associated with morbidity and long-term disability.
- Differences in clinical care and sociocultural factors cause that the evidence generated in high-income countries does not always translate to LAC region.
- It is a priority to develop comprehensive guidelines for optimum management and care within a wide variety of contexts and based on the specific conditions of the LAC region.

BRAIN INJURY IN LATIN AMERICA

The Latin America and Caribbean (LAC) consists of 33 countries with a population estimated at more than 590,000,000 and a large proportion of low- and middle-income countries (LMIC) with approximately 36% of the region's population living below the poverty line.[1,2] Cover an area that stretches from the northern border of Mexico to the southern tip of South America, including the Caribbean, containing widely different environments and consisting of many complex and heterogeneous ethnicities, societies, and cultures. Actually, approximately 30% of the population of LAC region do not have access to health care for economic reasons and 21% do not seek care

[a] Nursing Department, Universidad del Norte, Km 5 Via a Puerto Colombia, Área Metropolitana de Barranquilla, Colciencias 757, Barranquilla, Colombia; [b] Nursing Faculty, Universidad Nacional de Colombia, Av. Carrera 30 # 45-03 Ciudad Universitaria, Edificio 228, Enfermería, Bogotá, D.C., Colombia
* Corresponding author.
E-mail address: srortega@uninorte.edu.co

Crit Care Nurs Clin N Am 33 (2021) 101–107
https://doi.org/10.1016/j.cnc.2020.10.006
0899-5885/21/© 2020 Elsevier Inc. All rights reserved.

because of geographic barriers. Hence, a demographic, human and societal development has occurred in the last years.[1–4]

The LAC region has seen significant social and economic changes over the past 50 years. Nowadays, LAC region confronts 3 major demographic shifts: (1) population growth, (2) urbanization, and (3) aging; the population growth and aging are catching up with that of high-income countries and the 90% of the population now live in urban areas. The observed epidemiologic transition has led to an increase in risk factors and an increase in morbidity and mortality rates related to stroke. Of these risk factors, a significant proportion is attributed to classic preventable cardiovascular factors, such as hypertension and diabetes, but other modifiable factors also play a role, such as heavy alcohol consumption and smoking.[5] There are multiple causes of neurologic diseases that are endemic in Latin America, including neurocysticercosis, Chagas disease, malaria, hemorrhagic fever, Zika virus, and snake bites.

Acute neurologic injury, such as traumatic brain injury (TBI) and stroke, are an important cause of death and disability in LAC. As stated in the Global Burden of Disease 2016 Study (GBD 2016), neurologic disorders ranked as the leading cause group of disability-adjusted life years, years of life lost, and years lived with disability in Latin America.[6] Also, the impact of the disability is greatest in LAC due to several conditions that increase the risk and contribute to injury, such as the high use of motorcycles without helmets, speeding, drunk driving, and lacking seat belts, and the socioeconomic status that causes limited access to health care, unhealthy lifestyles, poor knowledge, and compliance with prevention strategies, increased stress, and underdiagnosis.[7]

For the prehospital, acute care and rehabilitation, according to Ouriques and colleagues the characteristics, models of health care systems, and prevalence of risk factors vary substantially across the LAC countries. Uruguay (58%) has the highest proportion of private health care systems and Argentina (8%), Guatemala (8%), Paraguay (7%), and Peru (7%) the lowest. Although 100% of the population in Argentina and Brazil and at least 90% of the population in Colombia, Costa Rica, and Panama are covered by the social security system, in Uruguay and Bolivia this coverage was available to only 37% to 65% of the population, respectively.[8]

Nevertheless, according to Avezum and colleagues[1] "the population is thereby getting better access to education, water and sanitation services, primary health care, technologies, and immunizations, as well as benefiting from sustained progress toward preventing and controlling numerous communicable diseases in several Latin American countries".

THE THREE DELAYS MODEL IN THE CARE OF PATIENTS WITH BRAIN INJURY

Mortality and morbidity mostly depend on the time required for patients to access care. Minimizing the time lost before care can be provided during the "golden hour" improves outcomes in patients with brain injury.[9,10] Several factors can delay the clinical assessment, management, and care of this patients especially in LAC region, and patients with acute neurologic conditions can deteriorate during these delays, contributing to the high rates of irreversible damage and death. Borrowing from the maternal health literature, the three delays model will be used to analyze this situation in Latin America and Caribbean.

First Delay: The Decision to Seek Care

The first delay represents time from injury to seeking care after an injury. For the acute neurologic injuries early access to the most appropriate medical treatment can improve health outcomes. Despite this, only 30% to 60% of people who experience a stroke seek medical help within the recommended 3-hour timeframe.[11] In TBI the situation is not much different; roughly 40% of the patients do not seek medical attention for their injury.[12] The 3 major reasons for not seeking care are discussed in the following section.:

Lack of recognition of the symptoms

In Latin America, the general population's knowledge of the term stroke is deficient. According to Diaz[13] and Scherle,[14] more than 70% of the subjects (patients and carers) admitted to having little knowledge or not knowing any alarm symptoms of stroke, which leads to thinking that the symptoms were not serious enough, and a lack of adequate response to its symptoms (delay in alerting the emergency department or in going to a health center). The most common reason given for not seeking medical care in patients with TBI is related to the thought that medical care is not necessary. Patients are less likely to seek medical care if they are older, suffer a mild TBI grade, or the injury occurs at home. Patients are more likely to seek medical attention if they are injured in a car accident, in a fall on the street, or experienced loss of consciousness or amnesia at the time of injury.[12] The severity of their symptoms is another characteristic in seeking care in both stroke and TBI. Severe or sudden rather than mild or slowly progressing symptoms are a significant motivator to direct the patients seek immediate medical attention.[15] As most of the injuries occur while riding in a car or motorcycle, patients and bystanders may recognize a critical injury and immediately seek care, whereas patients with milder injuries may not seek care until symptoms become more evident.[9]

Decision to first contact the nonemergency health services

This delay is strongly influenced by bystanders (family members, friends, neighbors, or work colleagues). Numerous factors affect whether bystanders are able to influence positively or negatively the patient's decision to seek help: the patient' s relationship with them, whether they were seen to have some "medical knowledge," their perception of the patient's ability to decide at that time, and their level of proactiveness in the situation. Bystander advice is associated with more rapid recognition and care.[16] A minority of bystanders delayed the help-seeking process. The reasons for this are not wanting to take responsibility for the decision but rather contacting someone else who they viewed was able to do it, perceiving the situation to be less urgent or serious, or misinterpreting the symptoms and thinking the situation was not serious.[17]

Financial, geographic, and cultural barriers

In Latin America an estimated 30% of the population has no access to health care for financial reasons, approximately 30% of Colombian users consider the price of consultations, drugs, and tests to be high at all care levels and 60% in inpatient care.[18,19] Roughly 21% is kept from seeking by geographic barriers[18] and long journey times to reach health services, and most of the time the injuries occur at night when the transportation is limited and more expensive, so patients and carers prefer to wait for the next day to seek care. Latin America people, particularly those from indigenous background, have an established history of using natural medicine. These traditions still hold strong in many parts of LAC today, providing many Latinos with a family custom of treating yourself without a professional doctor's help.

Second Delay: Reaching Care

The second delay is the time from the decision to seek care to the arrival at a hospital with capacity to manage. According to Calvello and colleagues[20] "the delay in identifying and reaching a medical facility depends on the planning and organization of prehospital emergency services" and requires change in nonhealth-sector policy, such as increased funding for infrastructure. Early identification and treatment of neurologic conditions in the prehospital sceneries improve outcome.[21] In Latin America prehospital care is less developed especially in LMIC, where utilization of formal emergency medical services is often very low.[7] The first responders are usually bystanders who recognize a critical injury and provide prehospital transport and occasionally first aid. The trajectory to the emergency department is frequently information relevant for the prognostic, such as pupillary examination and blood pressure. Studies in this field in LAC region do not draw conclusions about the influence of prehospital care in the patient's outcomes. More studies would provide valuable information that strengthen prehospital care in the region.

Third Delay: Received Care

Third delay is the time from arrival at the hospital to management by trained medical professionals.[9] Management of patients suffering from acute neurologic injury mandates high-quality care throughout; the goal for the management of the neurologic patient, once arrived to the hospital, is to stabilize and prevent secondary brain injury (SBI).[22] There are some aspects of acute care and SBI prevention that are still neglected in LMIC, resulting in a third delay: (1) patients are stabilized on arrival to the emergency department without a neurology/neurosurgery professional; the guidelines recommend that any patient with an urgent neurologic problem can be seen by a neurologist within 1 hour of the onset of symptoms; however, the times are around 0.2 and 3 hours or more[23]; (2) a bed in the intensive care unit for neuromonitoring may not be immediately available. During this delay, patients can neurologically deteriorate while they wait for care. The causes of third delay include many events along the path, from the arrival of an ambulance to the evaluation by a physician.[9]

Acute neurologic care

The countries in Latin America took longer than high-income countries to develop acute neurologic care. There were large variations in the delivery of acute stroke care among these countries. Some countries (eg, Bolivia, Ecuador, and Guatemala) still have few centers for acute stroke care, and even in countries with some level of organization to treat stroke (eg, stroke units, rehabilitation services), the quality of the services have to improve.[8] Stroke centers were available in LAC, although their number varied significantly between the countries. Whereas countries with few centers available are forced to transfer patients and find the hospital with the service, there are countries with various centers providing stroke care, which reflects the efforts by many physicians and hospitals to improve the quality of acute stroke management. Thrombolysis for patients with acute ischemic stroke was available in all countries, but only for a relatively small proportion of patients (less than 1%) the medication cost is often one of the reasons for not using thrombolytic therapy in patients with stroke in LMIC. An even smaller proportion of eligible patients received thrombectomy.[8]

Lack of neuromonitoring

The International evidence-based guidelines recommend use of intracranial pressure (ICP) monitors to assess and manage intracranial hypertension. However, ICP monitors and neuromonitoring are usually unavailable in LMIC and management of the patients remains based on imaging and clinical examination. Also no consensus-based/tested protocols or literature exists for acute brain injury treatment without ICP monitoring, and the only relevant literature on amenable protocols is based on the BEST-TRIP trial.[24] Beyond medical considerations, requirements for ICP monitoring include 2 principal considerations: (1) neurosurgeons are required to place the monitors; this is relevant in LMIC health system because the acute management is performed by critical care and physicians, and neurosurgical consultation is a limited resource; (2) most of the invasive monitoring systems are quite expensive, and in terms of prioritizing the resources, hospitals and health care systems choose to invest in more fundamental items with wider applicability to management in general.[24]

In spite of these situations, the received care met the requirements for high-complexity patients, and nurses are working hard every day to achieve favorable patient outcomes; reducing third delay is vital to reduce the morbidity associated with TBI and stroke and is known that it improved survival and reduced long-term disability.[9,12] In this scenario, it is a priority to develop comprehensive guidelines for optimum management and care within a wide variety of contexts and based on the specific conditions of the LAC region.[25]

THE LIFE AT HOME

The impact of an acute neurologic injury extends beyond the individual who has suffered a TBI or stroke. Returning home for survivors has increased and subsequently the burden to carers and other family members may be substantial.[26,27] Although the hospital level care received by all patients is appropriate and of good quality, the care received at home depended heavily on family resources and most of the population has several limitations to access to rehabilitation.[10] Most stroke and TBI survivors returning home under the care of family members are often unprepared for the caregiving role and lack training from health care providers. As a result, many family carers or care partners experience burden, depressive symptoms, and reduced health-related quality of life.[28]

Currently, the early supported discharge (ESD) from hospital to home has become a strategy to reduce hospital stay and complications. The implementation of this strategy should include an in-hospital–initiated intervention; nevertheless, this does not happen in most of the LAC countries and the "ESD" continues to be handled as the traditional standard care at discharge. Also, the interventions placed most of the highlighting on how to care for the survivor, rather than how to take care of oneself as a family carer. Future interventions should be designed to provide more emphasis on both patient's outcome and health and well-being of the family carer.

SUMMARY

Acute neurologic injuries are the leading causes of death and disability in Latin American countries. Currently, the absolute number of people with stroke and TBI, the number of people who survived, and the number of those who died have significantly increased. These data suggest that substantial problems exist in seeking care, reaching care, and receiving care including acute care and rehabilitation. The delays in the time between the symptoms onset and the time patient receives care increase the morbidity and long-term disability. Significant deaths and disability are found in LMICs due to increased risk factors, including a lack of prevention programs, low level of development of prehospital and hospital care for the patient with brain injuries, and the lack of rehabilitative services.[29] Differences in clinical care and sociocultural factors cause that the evidence generated in high-income countries does not always translate to LMICs, where the health infrastructure (including providers and facilities) is limited, creating a different context for care practice.[29] The applicability of high-income country clinical research standards and guidelines in LMICs is an important topic for future international research.

CLINICS CARE POINTS

- The major reasons for not seeking care in LAC region can be grouped in three: lack of recognition of the symptoms, decision to first contact with nonemergency health services and financial, geographic and cultural barriers.
- Mortality and morbidity in patients with brain injury mostly depend on the time required for patients to access care.
- Minimizing the time lost before care can be provided are vital to reduce the morbidity, long-term disability, and improved survival.

DISCLOSURE

The authors have nothing to disclose.

REFERENCES

1. Avezum Á, Costa-Filho FF, Pieri A, et al. Stroke in Latin America: burden of disease and opportunities for prevention. Glob Heart 2015;10(4):323–31.
2. Puvanachandra P, Hyder AA. Traumatic brain injury in Latin America and the Caribbean: a call for research. Salud Publica Mex 2008;50(SUPPL. 1):13–5.
3. Camargo ECS, Bacheschi LA, Massaro AR. Stroke in Latin America. Neuroimaging Clin N Am 2005;15(2):283–96.
4. Cantú-Brito C, Sampaio Silva G, Ameriso SF. Embolic stroke of undetermined source in Latin America. Neurologist 2017;22(5):171–81.
5. Soto Á, Peldoza M, Pollak D. Epidemiology and management of intracerebral hemorrhage in Chile. Aging - Life Span and Life Expectancy 2019. https://doi.org/10.5772/intechopen.86312.
6. Feigin VL, Nichols E, Alam T, et al. Global, regional, and national burden of neurological disorders, 1990–2016: a systematic analysis for the global burden of disease study 2016. Lancet Neurol 2019;18(5):459–80.
7. Ortega-Perez S, Sanchez-Rubio L, De las Salas R, et al. An international perspective of transition of neurological disease: the Latin american and the caribbean region. Nurs Clin North Am 2019;54(3):449–56.
8. Ouriques Martins SC, Sacks C, Hacke W, et al. Priorities to reduce the burden of stroke in Latin American countries. Lancet Neurol 2019;18:674–83.
9. Gupta S, Khajanchi M, Kumar V, et al. Third delay in traumatic brain injury: time to management as a predictor of mortality. J Neurosurg 2020;132(1):289–95.
10. Bonow RH, Barber J, Temkin NR, et al. The outcome of severe traumatic brain injury in Latin America. World Neurosurg 2018;111:e82–90.
11. Moloczij N, McPherson KM, Smith JF, et al. Help-seeking at the time of stroke: stroke survivors' perspectives on their decisions. Health Soc Care Community 2008;16(5):501–10.
12. Setnik L, Bazarian JJ. The characteristics of patients who do not seek medical treatment for traumatic brain injury. Brain Inj 2007;21(1):1–9.

13. Díaz R. Conocimiento de síntomas y factores de riesgo de enfermedad cerebro-vascular en convivientes de personas en riesgo. Acta Neurológica Colomb 2015; 31(1):12–9.
14. Scherle Matamoros CE, Rodríguez DR, San José ÁC, et al. Knowledge about ischemic stroke in Ecuadorian people. Rev Ecuatoriana Neurol 2018;27(3):44–50.
15. AL-Fayyadh S. Determinants of patient's decision-making in seeking care when experiencing stroke-associated warning signs. New Trends Issues Proc Humanit Soc Sci 2017;4(2):257.
16. Mellor RM, Bailey S, Sheppard J, et al. Decisions and delays within stroke patients' route to the hospital: a qualitative study. Ann Emerg Med 2015;65(3): 279–87.e3.
17. Zock E, Kerkhoff H, Kleyweg RP, et al. Intrinsic factors influencing help-seeking behaviour in an acute stroke situation. Acta Neurol Belg 2016;116(3):295–301.
18. Pan American Health Organization. Health financing in the americas. Available at: https://www.paho.org/salud-en-las-americas-2017/?p=178. Accessed March 28, 2020.
19. Garcia-Subirats I, Vargas I, Mogollón-Pérez AS, et al. Barriers in access to healthcare in countries with different health systems. A cross-sectional study in munic-ipalities of central Colombia and north-eastern Brazil. Soc Sci Med 2014;106: 204–13.
20. Calvello EJ, Skog AP, Tenner AG, et al. Applying the lessons of maternal mortality reduction to global emergency health. Bull World Health Organ 2015;93(6): 417–23.
21. Picinich C, Madden LK, Brendle K. Activation to arrival: transition and handoff from emergency medical services to emergency departments. Nurs Clin North Am 2019;54(3):313–23.
22. Zomorodi M, Brissie MA. Time is brain: setting neurologic patients up for success from emergency department to hospital admission. Nurs Clin North Am 2019; 54(3):325–33.
23. Soto V Á, Morales IG, Vega CC, et al. Tiempos de atención de urgencias neuro-lógicas en un hospital regional de alta complejidad. Rev Med Chil 2018;146: 885–9.
24. Hendrickson P, Pridgeon J, Temkin NR, et al. Development of a severe traumatic brain injury consensus-based treatment protocol conference in Latin America. World Neurosurg 2018;110:e952–7.
25. Johnson WD, Griswold DP. Traumatic brain injury: a global challenge. Lancet Neurol 2017;16(12):949–50.
26. McNair ND. The projected transition trajectory for survivors and carers of patients who have had a stroke. Nurs Clin North Am 2019;54(3):399–408.
27. Olson DWM, Juengst SB. The hospital to home transition following acute stroke. Nurs Clin North Am 2019;54(3):385–97.
28. Bakas T, McCarthy M, Miller E. An update on the state of the evidence for stroke family caregiver and dyad interventions. Stroke 2017;48(5):e122–5.
29. Iaccarino C, Carretta A, Nicolosi F, et al. Epidemiology of severe traumatic brain injury. J Neurosurg Sci 2018;62(5):535–41.

Moving?

Make sure your subscription moves with you!

To notify us of your new address, find your **Clinics Account Number** (located on your mailing label above your name), and contact customer service at:

Email: journalscustomerservice-usa@elsevier.com

800-654-2452 (subscribers in the U.S. & Canada)
314-447-8871 (subscribers outside of the U.S. & Canada)

Fax number: 314-447-8029

Elsevier Health Sciences Division
Subscription Customer Service
3251 Riverport Lane
Maryland Heights, MO 63043

*To ensure uninterrupted delivery of your subscription, please notify us at least 4 weeks in advance of move.

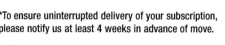